Implantable Bone Conduction Hearing Aids

Advances in Oto-Rhino-Laryngology

Vol. 71

Series Editor

G. Randolph Boston, Mass.

Implantable Bone Conduction Hearing Aids

Volume Editors

Martin Kompis Bern

Marco-Domenico Caversaccio Bern

74 figures, 42 in color, and 18 tables, 2011

KARGER

Basel · Freiburg · Paris · London · New York · Bangalore · Bangkok · Shanghai · Singapore · Tokyo · Sydney

Martin Kompis
Head of Audiology
Department of ENT, Head and Neck Surgery
University Hospital, Inselspital
University of Bern
CH-3010 Bern (Switzerland)

Marco-Domenico Caversaccio
Chairman and Director
Department of ENT, Head and Neck Surgery
University Hospital, Inselspital
University of Bern
CH-3010 Bern (Switzerland)

Library of Congress Cataloging-in-Publication Data

Implantable bone conduction hearing aids / volume editors, Martin Kompis, Marco-Domenico Caversaccio.
p. ; cm. -- (Advances in oto-rhino-laryngology, ISSN 0065-3071 ; v. 71)
Includes bibliographical references and indexes.
ISBN 978-3-8055-9699-2 (hard cover : alk. paper) -- ISBN 978-3-8055-9700-5 (e-ISBN)
1. Hearing aids. 2. Bone conduction. 3. Ear prosthesis. I. Kompis, Martin. II. Caversaccio, Marco-Domenico. III. Series: Advances in oto-rhino-laryngology ; v. 71.
[DNLM: 1. Hearing Aids. 2. Bone Conduction--physiology. 3. Hearing Loss--therapy. 4. Prostheses and Implants. W1 AD701 v.71 2011 / WV 274]
RF305.I47 2011
617.8'9--dc22

2011001118

Bibliographic Indices. This publication is listed in bibliographic services, including Current Contents®.

www.karger.com
Printed in Switzerland on acid-free and non-aging paper (ISO 9706) by Reinhardt Druck, Basel
ISSN 0065–3071
ISBN 978–3–8055–9699–2
e-ISBN 978–3–8055–9700–5

Contents

Audiological Aspects

Implantable and Nonimplantable Devices

Outlook

Preface

Since Anders Tjellström implanted and fitted the first patient with a bone-anchored hearing aid (Baha) in 1977, basic research and clinical work on implantable bone conduction hearing aids have advanced considerably. More adults and more children are implanted every year, up from only 3 in 1977 to a total of over 75,000 users today. An increasing number of centers all over the world offer implantable bone conduction hearing aids as one method of treatment. More knowledge is available than ever before. Better implants, more sophisticated signal processing and several designs from different manufacturers are available today.

Our aim was to bring together the most innovative, the most experienced, and the most renowned researchers and clinicians from all over the world to summarize current knowledge on implantable bone conduction hearing aids. Leading the center for implantable bone conduction hearing aids in Bern, which is the largest in Switzerland, we believe that this collection, which covers a wide range of relevant topics, will be useful for researchers and clinicians alike.

To meet this goal, this volume has been organized as follows. In Introduction and Basics, Anders Tjellström and Albert Mudry cover the history of bone conduction hearing devices, and Stefan Stenfelt gives an overview on acoustic and physiologic aspects of bone conduction hearing. The three following chapters describe three different systems which are available today. General surgical aspects are covered by a multicentered Swiss group of authors. Then, Ann-Louise McDermott from Birmingham and Jack J. Wazen from Sarasota, Fla., share their expertise on Baha in children and discuss complications of the procedure.

Different audiological aspects of implantable bone conduction hearing aids are covered in the next five chapters. Flurin Pfiffner reports on audiological results in different user groups in Bern, and the Nijmegen group summarizes current knowledge on binaural hearing with implantable bone conduction hearing aids. The group of John K. Niparko analyzes results of the growing number of patients who receive implantable bone conduction hearing aids because of their single-sided deafness, and our own group from Bern reports on the factors influencing the decision process in this group of patients and presents a new questionnaire. Mark Flynn from Cochlear, Inc., in Göteborg, Sweden, gives an update on digital signal processing for Baha.

A good knowledge of the alternatives to implantable bone conduction hearing aids is undoubtedly important, and therefore explored in the next two chapters. Andrzej Zarowski and colleagues from Antwerp explore headbands and softbands, and the Birmingham group compares different aspects of conventional hearing aids with implantable bone conduction hearing aids.

Make sure not to miss the very last chapter of this volume by Bo Håkansson on the future of

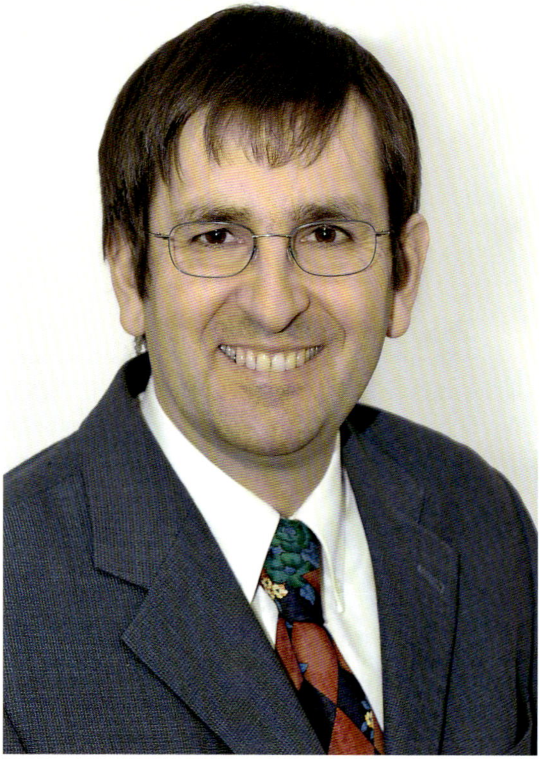

Martin Kompis

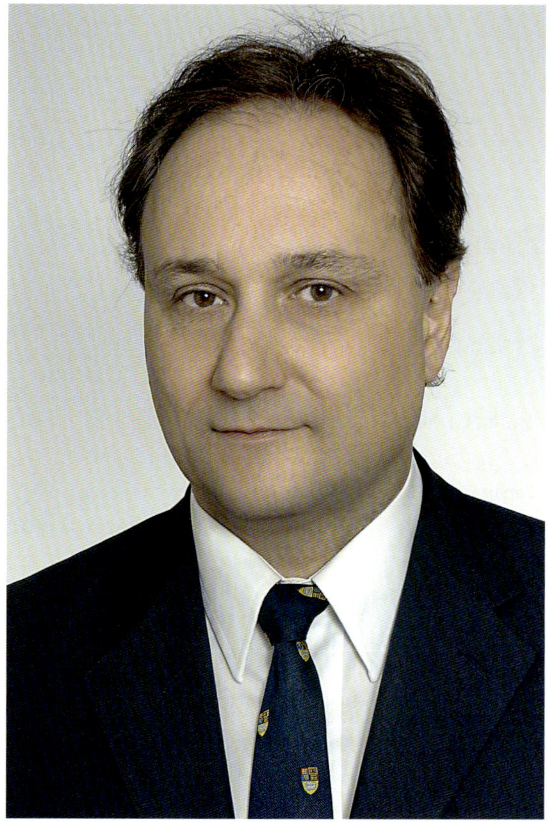

Marco-Domenico Caversaccio

bone conduction hearing aids; we promise a stimulating reading!

In a complex field such as implantable bone conduction hearing aids, manufacturers, clinicians and researchers contribute to successful development and the increasing patient benefit. In this volume, two chapters were contributed by researchers who are currently working for a manufacturer. Patrick Westerkull from Oticon, Inc., describes the Ponto system, and Mark Flynn from Cochlear has contributed an article on sound processing for Baha. Ralf Siegert, who reports on the Otomag system, describes himself as being close to the manufacturer.

We are very grateful for the high-quality chapters which have been contributed by experts from all over the world. We believe that this volume will be useful as a reference book for surgeons, audiologists, therapists, and people considering involvement with implantable bone conduction hearing aids. We hope you enjoy it.

Martin Kompis, Bern
Marco-Domenico Caversaccio, Bern

Kompis M, Caversaccio M-D (eds): Implantable Bone Conduction Hearing Aids.
Adv Otorhinolaryngol. Basel, Karger, 2011, vol 71, pp 1–9

Historical Background of Bone Conduction Hearing Devices and Bone Conduction Hearing Aids

Albert Mudry[a,b] · Anders Tjellström[c]

[a]Department Otolaryngology, Stanford University, Palo Alto, Calif., USA, and [b]Private Practice Lausanne, Switzerland;
[c]Department of Otolaryngology, Sahlgrenska Academy, University of Göteborg, Göteborg, Sweden

Abstract

During the last 20 years, bone-anchored hearing aids (Baha®) became a familiar solution in the treatment of some types of hearing loss. The aim of this chapter is to present the different historical steps which have permitted the production of this new bone conduction hearing device. The recognition of bone conduction hearing is old and was known at least in Antiquity. During the Renaissance, Girolamo Cardano demonstrated a method by which sound may be transmitted to the ear by means of a rod or the shaft of a spear held between one's teeth: this was the beginning of teeth stimulators to improve hearing, firstly in connection with a musical instrument and then, in the second part of the 19th century, with the speaker. The development of the carbon microphone at the beginning of the 20th century allowed the construction of the bone conduction vibrator placed on the mastoid area, notably supported by eyeglasses since the 1950s. Confronted by various problems, and notably the loss of part of sound in the soft tissue of the external mastoid, the idea to implant the vibrator into the mastoid bone was developed in Göteborg, and the first Baha was implanted in 1977 by Anders Tjellström. From that date, various improvements allowed the development of the actual Baha. These different steps are presented in this study, supported by original documentation.

During the last 20 years, bone-anchored hearing aids (Baha®) have become a familiar solution in the treatment of some types of hearing loss. Their technical development did not follow the giant steps of classical air conduction hearing aids during the last decades [1]. The idea to use bone conduction to improve hearing was not new, but nearly always unsuccessful. This was mainly in relation to the disadvantages associated with the necessary transcutaneous sound transmission to the skull bone. Part of the amplified sound energy was lost in the soft tissue especially in the high frequency range, so important for speech understanding in noisy surroundings. However, when reaching the bone of the skull the attenuation was small and level of distortion low. The major step in bone conduction hearing aid development was the possibility to have direct transmission to the bone with a rigid system implanted into it, i.e. the basic concept of the actual Baha. The aim of this chapter is to present the different steps which have allowed the production of these new bone conduction hearing devices.

Antiquity to Mid-19th Century

The recognition of bone conduction hearing is old and was known at least in Antiquity. It was assimilated to the sense of touch. In the 1st century, Pliny the Elder, a Roman scientist, remarked the potential of sound conduction through solid bodies, and he described the potential of bone conduction hearing in testing the flesh of some trees [2]. The Middle Ages did not bring forth anything new. During the Renaissance, Girolamo Cardano, an Italian physician, philosopher and mathematician, demonstrated a method by which sound may be transmitted to the ear by means of a rod or the shaft of a spear held between one's teeth: 'Here is a very surprising occurrence which everybody can experience. Place one end of a spear touching a lyre or even somebodies mouth, if another person then holds the opposite end of the spear between their teeth, as if hearing was present within the teeth, that person would hear distant sounds, voices and words that he could not hear under normal circumstances' [3]. Cardano described this experiment only as a curiosity rather than having practical value. At the same time, other scientists, such as Porta, Curaeus, Capivacci, Aquapendente, Plater and Ingrassia, also described this experiment. Giovanni Filippo Ingrassia, an Italian anatomist, presented the story of a man who became hard of hearing after an acute disease with obstruction of the external hearing canal. This patient was able to hear a guitar with as much pleasure as before, when he took the handle with his teeth or when he placed in his mouth a baguette which was touching the instrument by its other extremity [4]. It was Hieronymus Capivacci, an Italian physician, who first realized the clinical

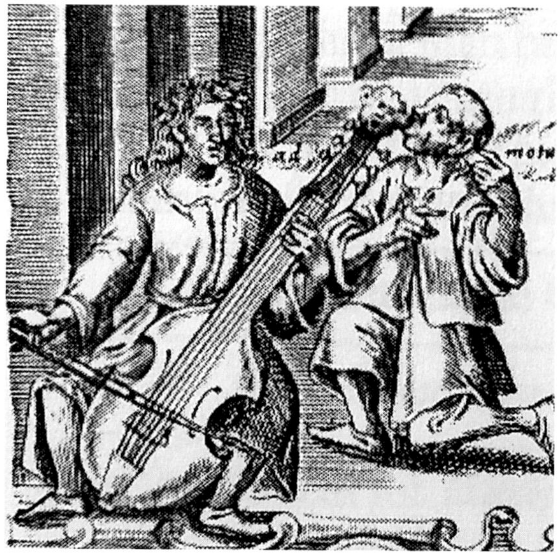

Fig. 1. Allegoric bone conduction by Bulwer in 1648.

significance of Cardano's experiment. He connected the teeth of a patient to the strings of a sitar by means of a 2 foot long iron rod. If the patient was able to hear sound from the sitar, a disease of the tympanic membrane was diagnosed, if he did not hear anything, it was a lesion of the auditory nerve [5].

Other scientists reported similar experiments during the 17th century, notably Cabeo, Kircher, Welsch, Sibscota, Riverius and Camerarius. Jakob Rudolf Camerarius explained that teeth had the same condition as the ear's ossicles, thus had the same possibility to transfer sound to the ear. Furthermore, the nerves of the teeth came from the nerve of the tongue which were in contact with the auditory nerves, thus explaining why when the sound reached the teeth, it was conducted on to the ear [6] (fig. 1). The 18th century, saw the same interest with the works of Trautmann, Boerhaave, Baumer, Jorissen, Haller, Buchner, Winkler, Buffon and Köllner [7]. In 1722, Christian Trautmann, a German senator then state judge, quoted an article or statement of Franz Christ Paullini regarding a man in Copenhagen who had lost his hearing due to distemper. By accident, this man found that by means of a stick of wood, he could understand the speech of others. For example, the man would place one end of the stick between his teeth and the other end just under the pulpit in a church, thereby understanding the speaker clearly [8]. Later John Paul Baumer [9], a young German physician, undertook to improve the device described by Trautmann. He used a rod of either glass, steel, copper, bell-metal, or silver, which was flat and broad at both ends. Baumer presented a young hearing-impaired lady who used an old rusty piece of sword blade, about 61 cm long, as a bone conduction appliance. Baumer also proposed using a speaking tube or a speaking trumpet as a bone conduction device via the teeth [10]. In 1757, Johann Jorissen [11], a German physician, published the first known dissertation dealing exclusively with hearing through the teeth [12]. Between 1799 and 1800, Vidron, a French master of music, invented a stick of steel, to improve the hearing of deaf persons. One end was placed on the table of the musical instrument and the other end between the teeth of the deaf person. Another branch, with a copper button on its end, was rested against the stomach and sometimes a third branch was placed on the skull. He presented his invention to the French Institute, which named some representatives to study the validity of this invention. Their investigations demonstrated that this system was not efficient for real deaf persons. Nevertheless, they tested the device by blocking their own external hearing canals and remarked that they heard better with the device. They concluded that this device could be good to treat hearing loss in relation with some kind of obstructions of the external hearing canal, and that it was ineffective for hearing loss originating in the auditory nerve or in relation to some 'essential internal trouble' [13].

In 1821, Jean-Marie Gaspard Itard, a French ear specialist, explained that sound was conducted through the bones of skull and developed one of the first bone conduction hearing devices: 'it is a sort of megaphone made of wood, pyramidal in form, with one side flattened like a whistle which should be held between the teeth of the deaf person. The other side ends in a horn, into which the person who is speaking places their mouth without touching it. The instrument must not be held but either suspended by a wire from the ceiling or held by a wooden fork placed on the floor. To make the instrument even more efficient, the walls should be very thick, at least two inches' [14]. To improve the quality of sound transmission, Itard proposed modifying the Jorissen system at the level of the end placed in the mouth of the speaker. Two ways of stimulation were then studied: by the teeth and later by the mastoid.

Teeth Stimulators

Even if hearing through the teeth had been a familiar phenomenon for a long time, it was only at the end of the 1870s that a number of new devices relying on teeth/bone conduction to air hearing were developed with great hope in the treatment of the deaf: The wonderful accuracy with which the phonograph and the telephone registered and reproduced the human voice, taken in connection with the fact that the nerves of hearing could be reached directly through the teeth and the cranial bones, led to the conclusion that if some instrument could be devised, sensitive enough to gather up the delicate sound vibrations that make up articulate speech, and convey them to the teeth, the problem of enabling the deaf to hear would be solved [15]. Following this concept, various instruments such as the Fonifero [16] (fig. 2), the Audiphone [17] (fig. 3), and the Dentaphone [18] (fig. 4) were developed [15]. These devices were essentially acoustic fans linked to the patient by a part held between the teeth. The Audiphone was tested in various schools for deaf persons [19], notably in France and the conclusion was 'that while for the many cases of partial deafness the Audiphone may replace the ear-trumpet, it does

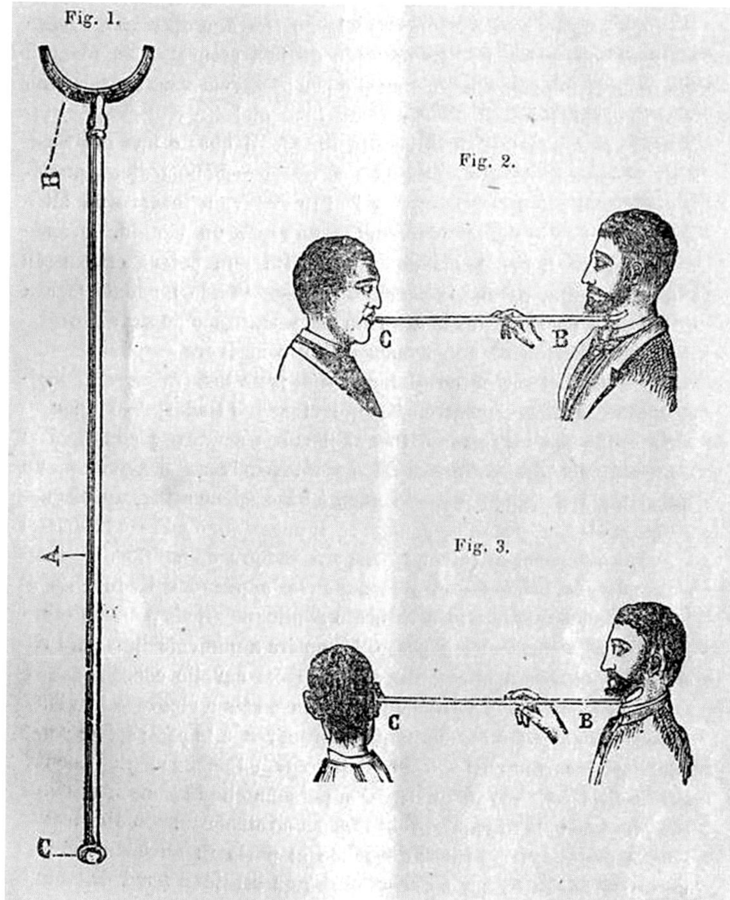

Fig. 2. Fonifero, 1876.

not, in its present shape, produce vibrations of sufficient force to be of much real service to the deaf-mutes' [20]. Such kinds of devices were already available at the beginning of the 20th century. The next step was to try to insert the device 'inside' the mouth.

In 1939, Albert Jefferis and Erwin Wilson patented another kind of Dentiphone for people with a denture. 'This invention relates to acoustics and more particularly to Audiphones and has for an object to provide means whereby persons having an attenuated sense of hearing may hear normal audible sounds. A further object of the invention is to provide a dentiphone built into and combined with a denture for use by persons having a hearing sense which is less than normal and who have also lost some of all of their natural teeth' [21]. The same year, Edmund Schwencke of New York patented a bone conduction receiver in a smoking pipe: 'A smoker's article having a stem adapted to be gripped by the teeth, said stem having a smoke passage there through, an acoustical vibrator unit mounted on said article, and a conducting rod operatively connected to said vibrator unit and extending through said stem, said rod being offset from said smoke passage and emerging from said stem to terminate outside of said stem at a point closely adjacent the position where

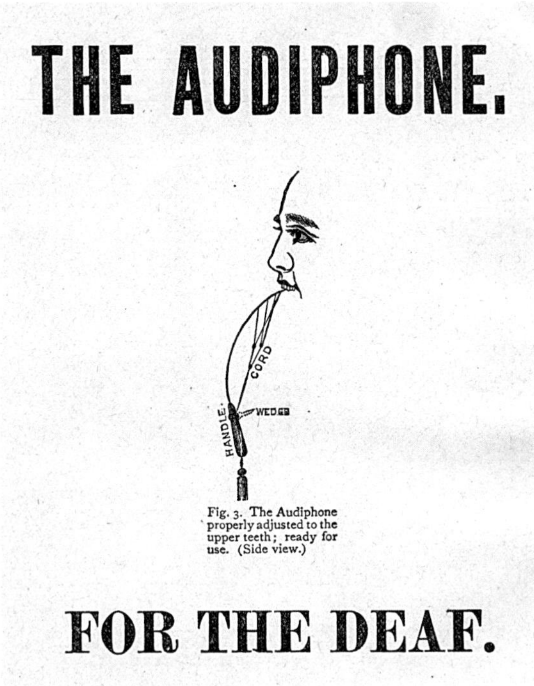

Fig. 3. Audiphone, 1879.

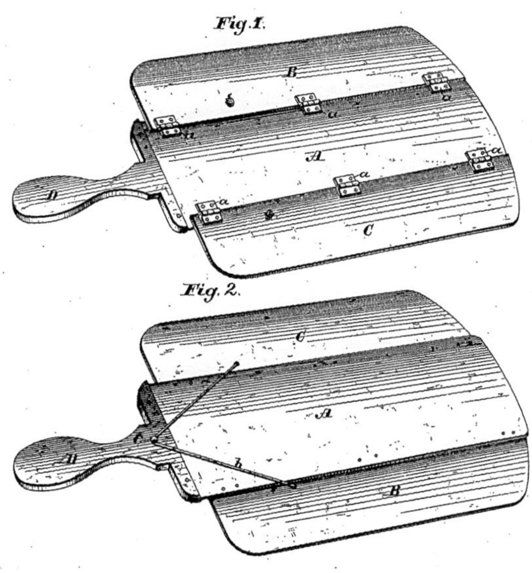

Fig. 4. Dentaphone, 1880.

said stem is normally gripped by the teeth in order that said rod may contact the teeth when the stem is so gripped' [22]. Other similar pipe devices were patented until 1961. The idea to stimulate bone conduction through the teeth was never abandoned [23].

Mastoid Bone External Stimulators

The development of the carbon microphone and the magnetic receiver (or earphone) at the beginning of the 20th century allowed the construction, in the beginning of the 1920s, of the bone conduction vibrator, also named oscillator. The primary difference was that the diaphragm of the receiver was connected to a metal or plastic plate or a small plunger to transmit the vibrations directly to the skull. In manufacture, the plunger or the plate was simply the bottom part of a small oblong or oval case which housed the magnetic assembly. In 1920, Joseph Prenn of Boston, patented a mechanical bone-conductive ear [24]. In 1925, Frederick Kranz, of Geneva, Illinois, patented the first real bone conduction vibrator (fig. 5). The objective was 'to provide an instrument by which alternating electric current either of a constant period or of the character of the usual telephone currents may be translated into mechanical vibration which can be transmitted to the bones of the subject' [25]. At first, the vibrator was held by a lorgnette handle so as to rest against the skull between the ear and the eyebrow, but soon they were held on a headband so as to make contact with the mastoid bone.

Bone conduction hearing devices found renewed interest amongst otologists when conductive hearing loss began being formally diagnosed. The advent of the bone conduction receiver held pressed against the mastoid eminence and its promulgation in 1931 and 1932 gave a tremendous impetus to the hearing aid industry. It remained for Hugo Lieber to develop, with the Sonotone Company, in 1933 [26], a small, wearable, bone

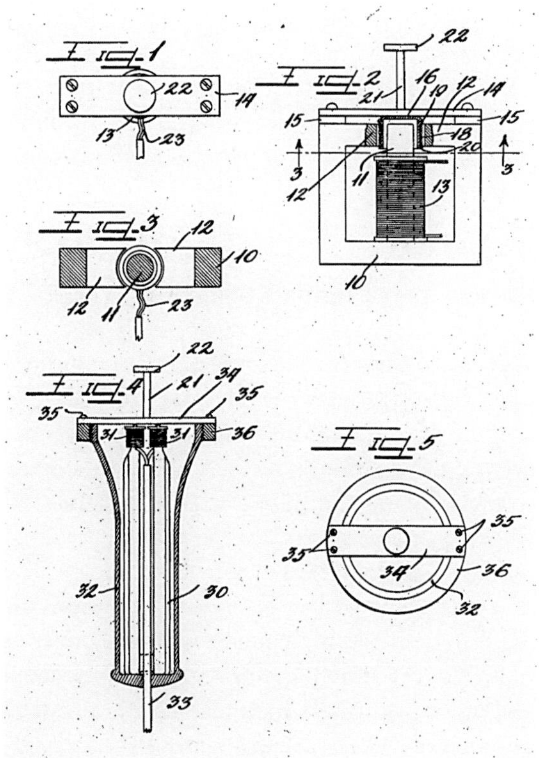

Fig. 5. Kranz's vibrator, 1925.

conduction receiver that could be adapted to the wearable carbon type hearing aid [27]. The most common type of bone conduction receiver was a magnetic receiver designed to vibrate its case instead of setting up sound waves in the air. The magnetic assembly being rigidly attached to a plastic case that is shaped to fit comfortably against the mastoid bone. Various other devices were then improved and produced. However, it was difficult to design a receiver that delivered high frequencies as efficiently as lower frequencies to the ear, partly because of the way skin and bone transmit sound [28]. The faster advancement of air conduction hearings aids as well as the public's greater familiarity with these devices caused most patients to prefer air conduction hearing devices over bone conduction devices despite a bone-conducting hearing aid being a better choice for a conductive hearing loss [29]. Another direction taken for the support of the hearing device was to fix it onto eyeglasses. Already used in 1909 [30], this idea was developed from the 1930s to the 1950s. In 1954 were introduced the first commercialized bone conduction eyeglasses by four different companies: Amplivox [31], Akumed [32], Otarion [33, 34] and Oticon. From the 1960s to the 1990s, bone conduction eyeglasses were the most widely used bone conduction hearing devices and then rapidly declined. Nevertheless, this idea lived on and continued to find scientists to improve the system at the turn of the 21st century [35].

Bone-Anchored Hearing Aid

Confronted by various problems, notably the part of sound lost in the soft tissue of the external mastoid, the idea to implant the vibrator into the mastoid bone began in Göteborg, Sweden, after the pioneer works of the anatomist Per-Ingvar Brånemark in bone rheology during repair phases [36]. He developed the concept of the osseointegration of a titanium metal screw in the bone. After extended animal experiments, the first clinical application was in the treatment of the edentulous jaw in 1965 [37]. In the mid 1970s, Brånemark tried to find a way to evaluate, acoustically, osseointegration in dental implants and discussed this with his ENT colleagues, notably Anders Tjellström. An Oticon bone vibrator was glued onto a snap coupling which was fitted to a dental implant, and then the arrangement connected to an audiometer. The patient reported that the sound was very clear and very loud, and it was necessary to turn the volume down to a very low level. With this montage, it was not possible to evaluate the degree of osseointegration, but it was clear that the sound propagated very well through the bones of the maxilla to the inner ear. This was one of the starting points for the future development of the hearing device Baha coupled with the titanium implant. Per Kylén,

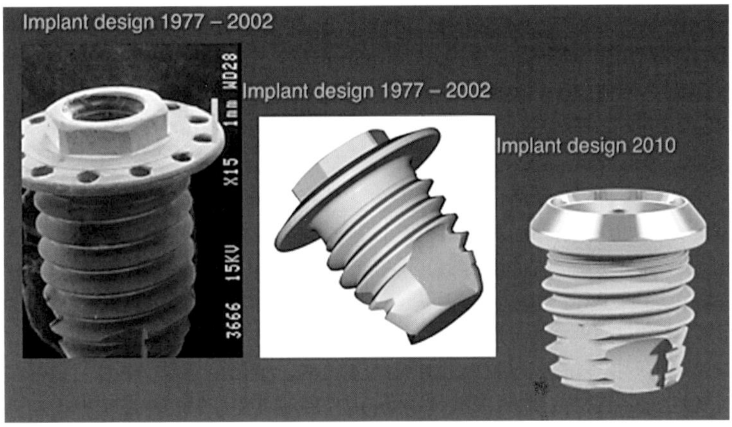

Fig. 6. First Baha implant in 1977.

another ENT colleague, who measured the noise levels at the otic capsule during mastoid drilling, based the second starting point on his findings [38]. He found that these levels were quite high, and in fact gave a temporary threshold shift, also indicating good sound transmission in bone. The third starting point was the dissatisfaction among patients with conventional bone conduction hearing aids with transcutaneous stimulation – discomfort, pain due to pressure, poor sound quality and a negative stigma.

In 1977, the first 3 patients (fig. 6) were fitted with implants for Baha, and the following year, another 10 patients [39]. All patients presented chronic ear disease in need of amplification but could not use air conduction hearing aids. The patients were followed carefully for 5 years, were very satisfied and no one lost his/her implant [40]. The implant and the special surgical instrument set were initially made by hand in Brånemark's workshop, but soon NobelPharma, later NobelBiocare, the company manufacturing the hardware for the dental implants took over the production. This company was, however, not interested in hearing rehabilitation, and in 1997 a new company, Entific, was formed with focus on the Baha hearing device and the implants for craniofacial rehabilitation. In 1983, another 23 patients were implanted, and in the following years between 30 and 60 new patients per annum.

The first international 3-day workshop on Baha was organized in Göteborg in 1986. Some 20 persons participated, thus launching its spread throughout the world. Among the 20 were David Proops from Birmingham, UK [41], and Cor Cremers from Nijmegen, the Netherlands [42]. Their institutions have treated more than 1,000 patients each and produced a great number of high-quality scientific papers. In 2005, Cochlear, a world leading corporation in cochlear implant technology bought the company and named it Cochlear Bone Anchored Solutions, located in Göteborg, thus giving a new impulsion to the production and development of new implants and new more sophisticated hearing devices. In September 2010, more than 80,000 are registered worldwide. Until 1989, the surgical procedure, based on a skin flap incision, to place the implant into the mastoid bone was a two-stage procedure to allow osseointegration without any load. This is still the routine in young children, but in adults a one-stage procedure [43] was then recommended and proven to be successful. Initially, no soft tissue reduction was performed, but it soon turned out that some of the patients experienced adverse skin reactions. In 1991, a new surgical technique based on a linear incision was proposed by the Nijmegen group.

In the same spirit, Jack Hough, Oklahoma City, USA, introduced, in 1981, another bone transducer, the Audiant. Using an orthopedic titanium screw for fixation, he placed a magnet in the mastoid process to osseointegrate. The external part held the other magnet for this electrodynamic transducer as well as electronics, microphone and battery. The test that Hough performed showed good fidelity and that it worked very well at threshold levels. However, in everyday life the output was too low. The main reason for this was that the distance between the two parts of the transducer was 6 mm with skin in between, making the magnetic field too weak to transmit the sound. The Audiant was on the market for a few years but is no longer available [44]. Following the concept of the Baha, Oticon showed new interest in direct bone conduction and produced their own system in 2009, i.e. a new titanium implant and a new hearing device.

Conclusion

The history of bone conduction hearing devices began in Antiquity. It was during the Renaissance that the phenomenon of bone conduction was first described, but it is only in the second part of the 19th century that the first bone conduction hearing devices, notably the Audiphone and the Dentaphone, were commercialized. Two main ways of stimulation were developed: through the teeth and through the mastoid bone [10, 45]. The mastoid was the preferred way, mainly with the invention of eyeglasses holding the hearing device on the mastoid region. The various proposed devices were not well tolerated and associated with different problems. Most of these problems were solved in the second part of the 20th century with the development of implantable devices fixed directly on the mastoid bone, such as the Baha.

References

1 Mudry A, Dodele L: History of the technological development of air conduction hearing aids. J Laryngol Otol 2000;114: 418–423.

2 Pliny: Natural history, vol IV. Loeb Classical Library. Cambridge, Harvard University Press, 2000, book XVI, LXXIII, p 507.

3 Cardano G: De subtilitate libri XXI. Parisiis, Fezandat & Roberri, 1550, liber XIII, p 234.

4 Ingrassia GF: In Galeni librum de ossibus dectissima et exspectatissima commentaria. Panormi, Maringhi, 1603, p 97.

5 Capivacci H: Opera omnia cura Johannis Hartmanni Beyeri. Francofurti, Paltheniena, 1603, Cap L, de laeso auditu, p 589.

6 Camerarius JR: Sylloges memorabilium medicinae et mirabilium naturae arcanorum centuriae 20. Tubingae, Cotta, Rommeius, 1683, Cap LXXI-LXXIV, p 102–104.

7 Panconcelli-Calzia: Das Hören durch die Zähne. Eine phonetisch-geschichtliche Vorstudie. Vox 1934;20:1–41.

8 Curtis JH: An essay on the deaf and dumb. London, Longman, Rees, Orme, Brown & Green, 1829, p 84.

9 Baumer JP: Prodomus methodi surdos a nativitate faciendi audientes et loquentes. Erfordiae, Hering, 1749, cap XI, p 9–10.

10 Berger K: Early bone conduction hearing aid devices. Arch Otolaryngol 1976;102:315–318.

11 Jorissen J: Dissertatio inauguralis medica sistens novae methodi, surdos reddendi audientes, physicas et medicas rationes. Halae Magdeburgum, Hendelianis, 1757, p 59.

12 Sonnenschein R, Leshin N: Functional examination of hearing. Arch Otolaryngol 1938;27:97–119.

13 Anonymous: Sur les moyens d'entendre par les dents. Bulletin des sciences, par la société philomathique de Paris. Paris, Fuchs, 1799–1801, vol II, p 133–134.

14 Itard JMG: Traité des des maladies de l'oreille et de l'audition. Paris, Maquignon, 1821, vol II, p 92–95.

15 Turnbull CS: The Audiphone and the Dentaphone. Arch Otol 1879;8:373–380.

16 Paladino G: Della transmissione fisiologica della voce atraverso le ossa del cranio merce il Fonifero, e del valore di questo nella clinica otojatrica. Movimento Med Chir 1876;8(331–332): 481–489.

17 Rhodes R: Improvement in audiphones. US Patent 219828.

18 Graydon T: Dentaphone. US Patent 225365.

19 Anonymous: The Audiphone. Am Ann Deaf Dumb 1880;25:95–96.

20 Anonymous: Aids to hearing. Am Ann Deaf Dumb 1880;25:225–228.

21 Jefferis A, Wilson E: Dentiphone. US Patent 2161169, June 6, 1939.

22 Schwencke E: Acoustical device. US Patent 2167377.

23 Popelka G, Derebery J, Blevins N, et al: Preliminary evaluation of a novel bone-conduction device for single-sided deafness. Otol Neurotol 2010;31: 492–497.
24 Prenn J: Mechanical bone-conductive ear. US Patent 1346721.
25 Kranz F: Vibration instrument for bone audition. US Patent 1540783.
26 Lieber H: Hearing-aid device. US Patent 1940553.
27 Watson L, et al: Hearing Tests and Hearing Instruments. Baltimore, Williams & Wilkins, 1949, p 277.
28 Davis H: Hearing and Deafness. A Guide for Laymen. New York, Staples, 1947, p 188.
29 Portmann M, Portmann C, Niclausse R: La prothèse électro-acoustique chez l'adulte. Rev Laryng (Bord) 1953;74: 68–97.
30 Rosenberg A: Means for effecting the cure or alleviation of deafness and other disorders of the auditory organs. GB Patent 190817138, August 12, 1909.
31 Berger K: The Hearing Aid. Its Operation and Development, ed 2. Livonia, National Hearing Aid Society, 1974, p 85.
32 Schumann E: Hörgerät fur Schwerhörige. Swiss Patent 315035, application October 2, 1952, received July 15, 1956.
33 Hollingsworth MH: Canadian Patent 666324. Spectacles concealed hearing-aid. US Patent 2930857, deposited December 31, 1953, accepted March 29, 1960.
34 Hollingsworth MH: Binaural hearing-aid device. US Patent 2930858, deposited July 15, 1954, accepted March 29, 1960.
35 Wandl R, Schermann K: Bone conduction hearing aid. US Patent 5673328, September 30, 1997.
36 Brånemark PI, Adell R, Breine U, Hansson BO, et al: Intra-osseus anchorage of dental prosthesis. Experimental studies. Scand J Plastic Reconstr Surg 1969;3:81–100.
37 Brånemark PI, Hansson BO, Adell R, Breine U, Lindström J, Hallén O, Öhman A: Osseointegrated implants in the treatment of the edentulous jaw. Experience from a 10-year period. Scand J Plat Reconst Surg 1977;16:1–132.
38 Kylén P, Arlinger SD, Bergholtz LM: Peroperative temporary threshold shift in ear surgery. An electrocochleographic study. Acta Otolaryngol 1977;84: 393–401.
39 Tjellström A, Lindström J, Hallen O, Albrektsson T, Brånemark PI: Osseointegrated titanium implant in the temporal bone. A clinical study on bone-anchored hearing aids. Am J Otol 1981;2:304–310.
40 Tjellström A, Rosenhall J, Lindström O, Hallen T, Abrektsson T, Brånemark PI: Five-year experience with skin-penetrating bone-anchored implants in the temporal bone. Acta Otolaryngol 1983;95:568–575.
41 Dutt S: The Birmingham bone anchored hearing aid programme. Some audiological and quality of life outcomes; thesis, Nijmegen, 2002.
42 Hol MKS: BAHA. New indications and long-term patient satisfaction; thesis, Nijmegen, 2005.
43 Tjellström A, Granström G: One stage procedure to establish osseointegration. A zero to five years follow-up report. J Laryngol Otol 1995;109:593–598.
44 Hough J, Himelick T, Johnson B: Implantable conduction hearing device: Audiant Bone Conductor. Ann Otol Rhinol Laryngol 1986;95:498–504.
45 Niemeyer W: Bone conduction hearing aids. Zeitschr Hör Akustik 1965;4: 194–204.

Albert Mudry, MD, PhD
Avenue de la Gare 6
CH–1003 Lausanne (Switzerland)
Tel. +41 21 3124333, Fax +41 21 3238325, E-Mail AMudry@ohns.stanford.edu

Kompis M, Caversaccio M-D (eds): Implantable Bone Conduction Hearing Aids.
Adv Otorhinolaryngol. Basel, Karger, 2011, vol 71, pp 10–21

Acoustic and Physiologic Aspects of Bone Conduction Hearing

Stefan Stenfelt

Department of Clinical and Experimental Medicine, Linköping University, Linköping, Sweden

Abstract

Bone conduction (BC) is the way sound energy is transmitted by the skull bones to the cochlea causing a sound perception. Even if the BC sound transmission involves several pathways including sound pressure induced in the ear canal, inertial forces acting on the middle ear ossicles and cochlear fluids, alteration of the cochlear space, and pressure transmission through the 3rd window of the cochlea, the BC sound ultimately produces a wave motion on the basilar membrane similar to that of air-conducted sound. The efficiency of the BC stimulation is largely dependent on the skull bone where the skull acts as a rigid body at low frequencies and incorporates different types of wave transmission at higher frequencies. The interaural stimulation difference is determined by the difference between contralateral and ipsilateral BC sound transmission: the transcranial BC sound transmission. To benefit from binaural processing, the transcranial transmission should be low, while the same should be high when using BC hearing aids for unilateral deaf subjects. By appropriately positioning the stimulation, high or low transcranial transmission can be achieved.

The conventional way of auditory stimulation is by an airborne sound that is transmitted through the ear canal, where it induces mechanical vibrations in the eardrum that are transmitted via the middle ear ossicles and become a sound pressure in the cochlea (scala vestibuli). This sound pressure acts on the basilar membrane producing a traveling wave that excites the sensory cells in the organ of Corti causing an auditory sensation. Bone conduction hearing is when the sound is transmitted through the skull bone, cartilage, skin and soft tissue, and fluids in the body, ultimately resulting in a sound pressure in the cochlear scalae. This type of sound transmission is sometimes divided between body conduction and bone conduction, where the latter is only sounds transmitted in the skull bone. Here, for simplicity, both body and bone conduction will be referred to as bone conduction and abbreviated BC.

Clinical Measurements using Bone Conduction

Understanding the processes of BC sound was early driven by its use for differential diagnosis between conductive and sensorineural hearing loss. In the 19th century, the usage of the tuning fork provided tests as Weber test and Rinne test [1]. After the introduction of the audiometer and the BC transducer (e.g. Radioear B71) during the 20th century, most diagnosis of conductive hearing losses is by comparison of air conduction (AC) and BC hearing thresholds (termed the air-bone gap). Although BC hearing thresholds are affected by an outer or middle ear lesion, the alteration is small compared to the change in AC thresholds, and the air-bone gap is often used to quantify the conductive loss.

It is sometimes desirable to use BC stimulation with other types of auditory measures such as speech recognition, otoacoustic emissions, or electrophysiology-based tests such as brainstem response audiometry [2–4]. Even if it is possible, the results are most often not directly comparable with those obtained using AC stimulation. This difference is mostly related to the difference in frequency response between earphones and the BC transducer, differences in hearing thresholds (sound pressure for AC stimulation and force for BC stimulation) and the general poorer dynamic range of a BC transducer (greater amount of nonlinear distortion). Moreover, testing setups for AC may be incompatible with BC excitation. An example of the latter is otoacoustic emissions [3], where normally the emissions are measured by a high-quality low-noise microphone tightly fitted in the ear canal giving a considerable occlusion effect, thereby affecting the result at frequencies below 2 kHz (see later section) [5].

The most commonly used BC transducer for audiometry is the Radioear B71 which has well-known characteristics and is used in the international standard for hearing thresholds [6]. The drawback of this device is poor dynamic and frequency range: the great amount of nonlinear distortion and housing resonances limits its practical use to the frequency range 0.25–4 kHz and levels below 60–70 dB HL. These limitations have often been addressed, and recently another BC transducer was proposed enabling high-frequency BC testing [7]. Other designs of BC transducers providing greater dynamic range [8] and measurement of the transducer-skull interface [9] have also been suggested to improve BC audiometry.

Basilar Membrane Stimulation

One important issue related to perception of BC sound is the sensory input to the neural system. Since BC vibration causes motion of the whole skull and, most probably, also other parts of the human body, the vibration perception is not necessarily only auditory. At lower frequencies and at higher stimulation levels, BC sound causes vibrotactile excitation and the perception is multimodal [10]. Moreover, BC vibration stimulation can excite the vestibular system, which is especially noticeable in large vestibular aqueduct syndrome and semicircular canal dehiscence [11]. In a study on loudness growth comparing AC and BC sound, it was shown that the loudness of BC sound increased more compared with loudness of AC sound, especially at the low frequencies [12]. This may be explained by multimodal excitation when stimulation is by BC resulting in a greater growth of loudness compared to AC sound for equal increase in sound intensity.

It is well established that BC sound perception is primarily caused by basilar membrane vibration. Firstly, BC pure tones can be cancelled by AC tones [13–15], indicating that the two ways of stimulation excite the same sensory cells for auditory perception. Secondly, direct measurement of basilar membrane motion shows similar excitation pattern independent of whether stimulation is by AC or BC [16]. Thirdly, electrophysiology measures such as brainstem audiometry give similar results for AC and BC stimulation when differences in stimulation spectrum are corrected for [17] and, fourthly, distortion product otoacoustic emissions can be generated by one AC and on BC tone [3]. Even if a BC sound influences the whole cochlea and not only a local point as AC sound, the inherent response of the basilar membrane is always a wave motion beginning at the base

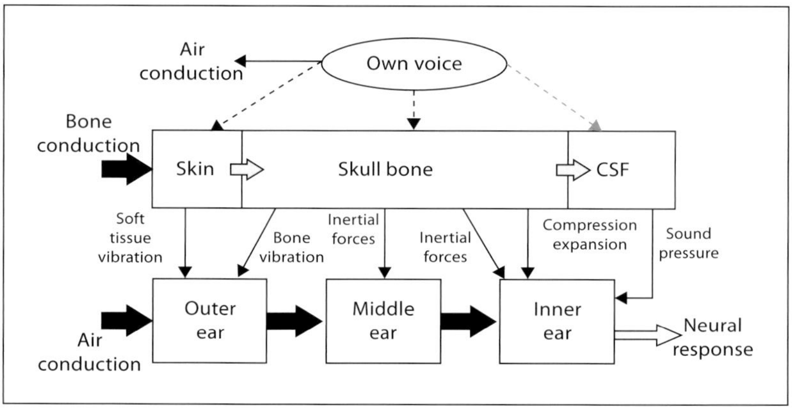

Fig. 1. A model of the pathways for hearing BC sounds. A BC vibration on the compressed skin of the skull bone causes vibrations of the skull and also produces a sound pressure in the skull interior. The vibration of the skin and bone produces a sound pressure in the ear canal, while inertial forces cause relative vibration between the ossicles and the surrounding bone. The sound is transmitted to the inner ear from the outer and middle ear, but also directly through inertial forces acting in the cochlear fluids, through compression and expansion of the cochlear space, and, to some extent, through sound pressure transmission from the skull interior. The own sound production is transmitted to the inner ear by both airborne sound and BC.

traveling towards the apex [18]. Therefore, the assumed important parameter for BC-induced wave motion on the basilar membrane is the pressure difference between scala vestibuli and scala tympani.

Pathways for Bone-Conducted Sound

Since it became generally accepted that humans can perceive BC sound, theories of how a BC vibration in the skull bone becomes a basilar membrane vibration have been presented. Early theories identified one or two pathways that resulted in BC sound. Today, it is generally accepted that BC sound transmission involves multiple pathways, and there is no obvious way to distinguish between them. One often used categorization is the anatomical division where BC sound affecting the outer, middle, and inner ear is referred to as the outer ear component, the middle ear component, and the inner ear component, respectively [19]. However, this categorization does not divide between different physical processes that are involved in the transformation from a skull bone vibration to a pressure difference between scala vestibuli and scala tympani and subsequent basilar membrane wave motion. Tonndorf [20], who investigated different mechanisms contributing to BC sound perception in the cat, identified seven components believed to be important for BC sound. In a previous paper, five components were presented as the most important for BC sound perception in the normal and impaired ear [21]. Below is a short summary of these five components (fig. 1).

Sound Pressure in the Ear Canal and the Occlusion Effect

When the skull is excited with BC sound, the ear canal deforms due to the vibrations, and airborne sound is produced in the ear canal. This sound is transmitted to the eardrum and further transmitted through the middle ear ossicles and produces a sound pressure in the scala vestibuli causing a basilar membrane traveling wave. Consequently, this BC sound pathway is similar to an AC sound transmission and should be considered as a skull vibration-produced AC sound. This means that this pathway is affected by the status of the outer and middle ear and the transmission is altered by it. For the normal open ear, the contribution of the ear canal pathway of BC sound is some 10 dB below other contributors at frequencies below 2 kHz and less important at higher frequencies [22]. The outermost part of the ear canal comprises cartilage and soft tissue, and is referred to as the cartilage part of the ear canal, while the innermost part is surrounded by skull bone known as the bony ear canal. If the BC transducer is positioned close to the ear canal, for example on the mastoid, the soft tissue is efficient in transmitting the sound to the ear canal at low frequencies, while the bony part is the primary source for the BC-induced ear canal sound pressure at higher frequencies [22].

The outer ear pathway of BC sound can be dominating at lower frequencies if the open part of the ear canal is closed, often termed the occlusion effect. The effect of occluding the ear canal depends on the type and position of the occluding device, but can give up to 40 dB increased sensitivity to BC sound at low frequencies [5]. The origin of the occlusion effect is the change in radiation impedance at the ear canal opening. With the ear canal open and at low frequencies, the radiation impedance is low, and a large part of the sound energy induced in the ear-canal by the BC skull vibration leaks out of the ear canal. However, if the canal is occluded, the sound energy is trapped and transmitted to the eardrum. This phenomenon was described by Tonndorf [20] and later modeled in Stenfelt and Reinfeldt [5]. As predicted by von Békésy [23], the model showed that if the occlusion is deep enough, the occlusion effect is insignificant [5]. Also, if circumaural devices are used, the enclosed volume is primarily determining the occlusion effect where greater volume results in less occlusion effect. It should be noted that the occlusion effect measured as change in ear canal sound pressure is usually 5–10 dB greater than the occlusion effect as measured by alteration of BC hearing thresholds at frequencies below 1–2 kHz [5].

Inertia of the Middle Ear Ossicles

From a mechanical point of view, the middle ear ossicles are suspended in the middle ear space by the eardrum, ligaments, and tendons. Most important for BC sound is the eardrum and the annular ligament positioning the stapes footplate in the oval window: these two act as mechanical springs attached to the free masses (ossicles). When the skull bone surrounding the middle ear cavity vibrates due to BC excitation, the spring effect causes the ossicles to vibrate in phase with the skull at low frequencies. At higher frequencies, the ossicles become vibrationally decoupled from the surrounding bone resulting in a relative motion between the stapes footplate and the otic capsule. This behavior was experimentally verified in Stenfelt et al. [24], where the ossicles vibrated with the surrounding bone at low frequencies and showed large relative motion above the middle-ear ossicle resonance frequency of 1.5 kHz. This finding was later verified in Homma et al. [25] showing that the difference in middle ear ossicle resonance frequency between BC and AC [e.g. 26] sound was caused by differences in vibration modes of the ossicles.

It has been speculated that the middle ear ossicle inertia is important for BC sound perception at frequencies around the resonance frequency and below, i.e. approximately 2 kHz and below. Supporting this theory is, for example, the worsening in BC thresholds around 2 kHz following immobilization of the ossicles due to otosclerosis of the stapes (also known as the Carhart's notch) [27] and increased BC sensitivity below 2 kHz with artificial mass loading of the ossicles (lowering the resonance frequency) [28]. When comparing ossicle vibration at hearing threshold with AC and BC stimulation, it was found that the ossicle inertia can be important for BC perception in the normal ear at and slightly above the resonance frequency (2–3 kHz) [29].

Inertia of Cochlear Fluids and Fluid Pressure Transmission

The fluid in the cochlea is also subject to inertial forces when the bone surrounding the cochlea vibrates. The result of these forces is a pressure gradient across the basilar membrane that would form a traveling wave. Since the fluid can be considered incompressible, a fluid flow in the cochlea would require compliant inlet and outlet of the fluid on both sides of the basilar membrane. The two obvious examples are the oval window on the scala vestibuli side and the round window on the scala tympani side. However, there are several other structures that can act as compliant pathways of the cochlea. These structures are collectively known as the third window [30]. This means that, as long as there is a pressure gradient over the basilar membrane, there will also be fluid flow acting on the basilar membrane initiating a traveling wave.

The pathways other than the oval and round windows that enable pressure and fluid transmission to and from the cochlea include the vestibular and cochlear aqueducts, nerve fibers, veins, and micro-channels entering the cochlea [31]. It has for example been noticed that an improved fluid connection between the vestibular space and the cranial space, known as a semicircular canal dehiscence, improves the low-frequency BC sensitivity [11]. Similar results are found when the dehiscence is made artificially into the middle ear space [32]. The concept of the third window offers two different interpretations of BC stimulation pathways. One is the inertial effects of the cochlear fluid resulting in a fluid displacement mentioned above. The other interpretation is sound pressure transmission from the cranial space to the cochlea [33]. It has been shown that static pressure can be transmitted from the cranial space to the cochlea [34]; the same is also possible for dynamic pressure [33]. This type of transmission has primarily been attributed to a patent cochlear aqueduct, but the vestibular aqueduct and other channels may well enable such mechanism. Although the sound pressure transmission from the skull interior to the cochlea has been suggested as an important BC contributor, clinical results as transcranial transmission and pathological findings in semicircular canal dehiscence and large vestibular aqueduct syndrome suggest that this contributor to BC sound perception is not the most important one.

It has been estimated that only a small fraction of the fluid of the cochlea (less than one millionth) is necessary to be displaced to give a hearing sensation of 80–100 dB HL [21]. This indicates that the fluid inertia would be an efficient way to excite the cochlea. Moreover, in cases of immobilization of the stapes, e.g. otosclerosis of the stapes, the AC hearing thresholds deteriorate significantly while the BC thresholds are only slightly affected in the 2 kHz range. Since transmission through the middle ear is severely reduced in such case, the BC sound is transmitted directly to the cochlea. Moreover, the skull is believed to constitute near-rigid body motion (wavelength longer than the size of the skull) at lower frequencies, compression and expansion of the cochlear walls cannot explain the BC sound perception. Consequently, for lower frequencies, fluid inertia is likely the most important pathway for BC sound in the normal ear but probably less important at higher frequencies.

Alteration of the Cochlear Space

When a transversal wave propagates in the skull bone, the skull bone compresses and expands with the wave. This means that the structure deforms. When such wave affects the cochlea, the deformations alter the cochlear space, causing a fluid motion that gives a sound pressure. This pathway was termed inner ear compression by von Békésy [19] and distortional component by Tonndorf [20], and has often been central when explaining BC sound perception. The theory for the compressional response is that the cochlea is unsymmetrical regarding scala tympani and scala vestibuli. Scala vestibuli space is about 50% greater than scala tympani, and the impedance of the oval window is greater (stiffer) than the impedance of the round window (more compliant) [20]. Consequently, when the cochlea is compressed, excess fluid is forced from the scala vestibuli side to the scala tympani side and the round window. The opposite happens when the cochlea expands, i.e. fluid flows from scala tympani towards scala vestibuli, thereby exciting the basilar membrane.

The cochlea is coiled, and its dimension can be thought of like a sphere with approximately 10-mm diameter. If the limit for effective compression response is set to a wavelength that is less than ten times the size of cochlea, the lowest frequency where the compressional response would be an effective excitation of the cochlea would be 4 kHz. This is in line with other estimations of its importance in the normal ear of the human [21].

Bone Conduction Sound Transmission in the Skull

The human cranial bone comprises dense cortical bone with fluid-filled spondaic bone in between, loaded on one side with skin and subcutaneous tissue and fluid (cerebrospinal fluid) and brain tissue on the other. Also, the bone in the skull base, where the inner ear is situated, differs from the cranial bone with thicker and denser bone structure. To complicate things even more, the skull is not a single bone structure but consists of several parts fused with sutures. Due to its complexity, modeling efforts have so far only provided limited insight to the BC sound transmission in the skull.

Most earlier experimental studies of BC sound transmission focused on the motion of the skull surface [19, 35, 36], while more recent studies have measured the response at the cochlea, either in all three space dimensions [37, 38] or in one dimension [39, 40]. Even if these studies provide insight into the vibration characteristics of the skull bone and differences in transmission efficiency between stimulation positions and the cochlea, it is not clear how to relate a vibration of the cochlea to a hearing sensation. However, the hypothesis is that, in relative terms, a greater vibration response of the cochlea at a specific frequency leads to a greater BC sound perception. It was shown in the Stenfelt and Goode study [38] that with BC stimulation at the skull surface, the cochlea vibrates in all space dimensions without any dominant direction.

In normal BC hearing testing, the BC transducer is placed on the compressed skin that transmits the BC vibration to the skull bone. The effect of the skin, in terms of dynamic force transmission, is small at low frequencies but will attenuate the BC sound at frequencies above approximately 2 kHz [41]. Moreover, the transmission through the skin improves with the area of the skin transducer interface and static pressure between transducer and skull [14]. If the vibration transducer is coupled directly to the skull bone, as with the bone-anchored hearing aid [42] coupling system, the attenuation caused by the skin is avoided. For hearing testing, the attenuation of BC sound through the skin can often be overcome by an increase in the output from the audiometer. For BC hearing aids, where the output is limited, the skin attenuation is of greater importance. Since the attenuation depends on both the BC hearing aid design and the skin and skull impedance, a specific number for this skin attenuation cannot be given. But, a general 5- to 15-dB improvement in sensitivity at frequencies above 1 kHz can be expected when the BC transducer is attached directly to the skull (as with the bone-anchored hearing aid) instead of the compressed skin.

A general finding is that the closer the stimulation position is to the cochlea, the greater the

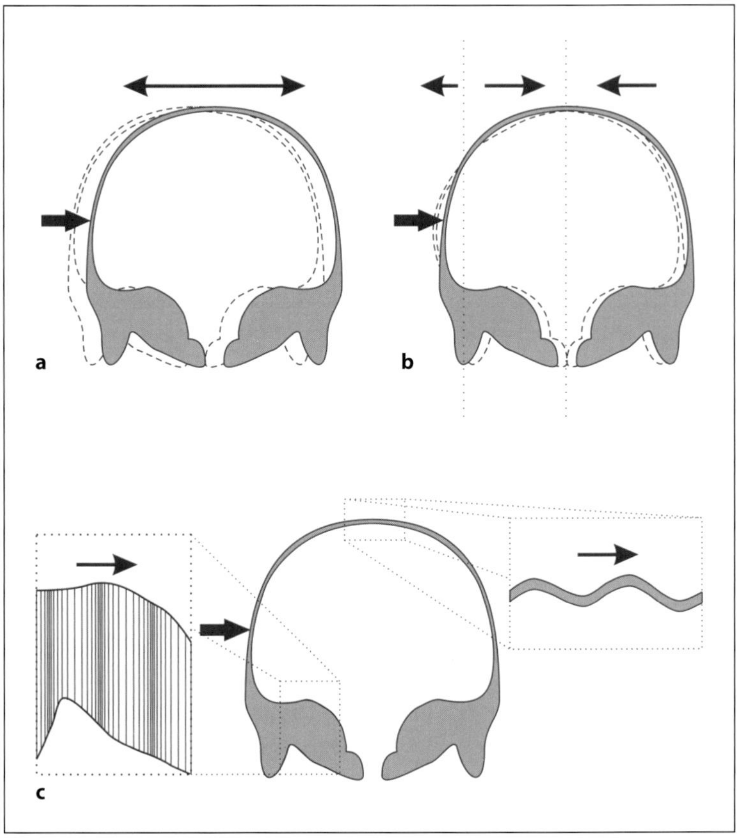

Fig. 2. Illustration of the vibration modes of the human skull for frequencies between 0.1 and 10 kHz. For simplicity, the vibrations are shown as one-dimensional motions, while the real human skull shows vibration responses in all space dimensions. The thick arrows indicate the stimulation position, and the thin arrows indicate the response directions. The rigid body response at the lowest frequencies is illustrated in **a**, while the mass-spring system response at frequencies between approximately 0.3 and 1.0 kHz is shown in **b**, where three sections of the skull move sequentially in opposite directions. **c** The vibration responses for frequencies above 2 kHz are illustrated differently for the skull base and the cranial vault. At the skull base, longitudinal wave propagation dominates the response, while a mixture of vibration modes including bending waves is present at the cranial vault.

BC sound stimulation of the cochlea. This is frequency dependent, and the greatest improvement is seen at the highest frequencies [38, 40]. In a study investigating the squamosal suture's influence on BC sound transmission, an average attenuation of about 2 dB was found for frequencies above 2 kHz [40]. However, it could not be concluded if the attenuation was a pure effect of the suture, of moving the stimulation position closer to the cochlea, or a combination of both.

The vibration modes of the skull have been reported in several studies [e.g. 19, 38], and for the frequency range 0.1–10 kHz four different types of vibration modes appears (fig. 2). At the very low frequencies, below the resonance frequency of the skull mechanical point impedance (150–400 Hz), the skull behavior can be approximated with rigid body motion (fig. 2a) [38]. Above this region and up to about 1 kHz, where the first global skull resonance appears [35], the skull vibration can be described as a mass-spring system, where large parts of the skull move in phase (e.g. the petrous part of the temporal bone hosting the cochlea; fig. 2b). Above 1 kHz, wave transmission appears in the cranial bone, and between 1 and 2 kHz the skull transitions from a mass-spring-like behavior to be dominated by wave transmission. The wave transmission types differ between the cranial vault and the skull base (fig. 2c), where the wave speed in the skull base seems constant at approximately 400 m/s, while the wave speed in the cranial vault is frequency dependent with around 250 m/s at 2 kHz increasing to 300 m/s at 10 kHz [38].

Transcranial Transmission

The BC stimulation at one mastoid is transmitted to both cochleae, and for testing BC thresholds the non-test ear requires masking to ensure the response from the test ear. For simplicity, in audiometry the BC sound transmission to the contralateral cochlea is often assumed equal to that of the ipsilateral cochlea (transcranial transmission equals 0 dB). However, there can, at certain frequencies, be substantial interaural differences of up to 40 dB, where the sound is either greatest at the ipsilateral or the contralateral cochlea [43]. When BC sound transmission is estimated from vibration measurements at the cochlea, the transcranial transmission is close to 0 dB for frequencies up to 1 kHz, where it starts to decrease and becomes –15 to –20 dB at 10 kHz [38, 39].

We measured the transcranial transmission in 30 unilateral deaf subjects using both the normal mastoid stimulation position for BC audiometry and the typical BAHA implant position some 55 mm behind the ear canal opening in the parietal bone. Bone-conducted hearing thresholds were obtained at 31 1/6th octave frequencies between 250 Hz and 8 kHz. From these data, it could be concluded that there is a general trend of greater interaural differences at the higher frequencies (fig. 3). However, the individual spread was great, and no general trends in the specific configuration of the transcranial transmission were found. It was also seen that a normal audiometric positioning of the BC transducers gave greater interaural differences than a positioning at the usual BAHA implant site. According to Eeg-Olofsson et al. [39], the transcranial transmission is almost independent of the position of the contralateral stimulation transducer. When transcranial transmission (or the opposite, transcranial attenuation) is measured as the difference in sensitivity between a contralateral and ipsilateral stimulation at symmetrical positions, it is the ipsilateral transmission that dominates the interaural difference.

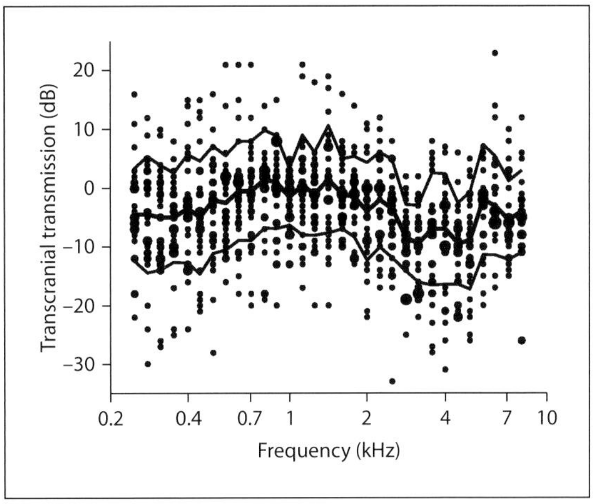

Fig. 3. Transcranial transmission of BC sound measured as the ipsilateral sensitivity related to the contralateral sensitivity when stimulation is on the mastoid (normal BC audiometry position). A positive number indicates better transmission from the contralateral side. The dots indicate individual results (a larger dot indicates several individuals with equal result). The thick solid line (in the middle) is the median of all subjects, and the thinner solid lines are the median ± 1 standard deviation.

From the perspective of BC hearing aids, a low transcranial transmission (i.e. the stimulation of the ipsilateral cochlea is substantially greater than the contralateral cochlea) is beneficial when bilateral application is used since more binaural information can be extracted from the two stimulation positions (less cross-over transmission, see below). However, from the perspective of using BC hearing aids for unilateral deaf subjects, a high transcranial transmission is beneficial as more BC sound energy is transmitted from the deaf side to the healthy cochlea.

Binaural Bone Conduction Hearing

Binaural auditory processing are functions that are superior by the use of two ears rather than one including the ability to localize sound sources in three dimensions and identify speech in a noisy environment. The general understanding is that the human uses interaural temporal differences at frequencies below 1 kHz and interaural level differences at the higher frequencies for efficient binaural processing. Both the temporal and level differences can be negatively affected by the BC transcranial transmission reducing the information separation between the cochleae. The low temporal differences between the cochleae at low frequencies with BC sound shown in Stenfelt and Goode [38] impede the low-frequency binaural processing. At the high frequencies, the transcranial transmission may limit the level separation normally given by the head shadow; this could also impede binaural processing. So how efficient is bilateral application of BC sound in terms of binaural hearing, for example with BC hearing aids?

It should be noted that the following discussion is limited to two rather similarly functioning cochleae; binaural auditory processing is not possible for unilateral profound deaf subjects. The research into BC binaural hearing is sparse and has mainly been directed to binaural benefit in patients with bilaterally fitted BAHA [44, 45]. Those studies have shown that there are benefits in terms of better spatial perception (sound localization) and release of masking for bilateral BAHA users compared with monaural application. Also, studies in normal hearing subjects have indicated similar results: there are binaural benefits with bilateral BC stimulation, but the binaural processing is not as good as when then the stimulation is purely by AC [46, 47]. One way to quantify the binaural processing ability with BC stimulation has been to measure binaural masking level differences using low-frequency sinusoids in narrowband masking noise [44, 45]. Besides the binaural masking release, the stationary sinusoids from the two sources add constructively or destructively depending on the signal phases, and the results are influenced by the summation of two signals as well as of binaural effects: these cannot be separated [39]. Consequently, the binaural masking level differences test using stationary sinusoids is not suited for testing binaural processing with BC stimulation.

Own Voice

Most people are familiar with the influence of BC on their own voice: when listening to a recording of one's own voice, people are often struck by the difference between the recording and the way they normally perceive their own voice. The difference is that while the recording only picks up the airborne sound, we hear ourselves through both AC and BC sound (see fig. 1). The importance of the two pathways of our own voice, AC and BC, have been estimated by von Békésy [48] to be approximately equal; it was later estimated that the AC component is most important at low and high frequencies, while the BC component dominated the own voice between 0.7 and 1.2 kHz [49]. A recent thorough investigation showed large differences in the AC and BC components for 10 speech sounds [50]. It was concluded that the differences originated in the sound production itself; sounds that are produced similarly and belong to the same speech sound groups had similar relation between AC and BC contribution of one's own voice. Even if later studies confirmed von Békésy's result of approximately equal proportion of AC and BC sound for own voice perception, they also showed frequency dependency between the pathways as a function of the sound produced [49, 50].

It has been argued, for example by Bárány [51], that own-made sounds such as vocalization, chewing, etc., are less in animals with three middle-ear ossicles than in animals with only one bone. Due to the three-bone structure, the effective mass, and consequently the inertial force, are less than in a single-bone structure. As a result, the influence of the middle ear ossicle inertia is lower. Also, the stapedius muscle is elicited during vocalization [52]. Such contraction affects the low-frequency sound transmission through the middle ear. It would also impede inertial force effects on the middle ear ossicles. However, to what extent the stapedius muscle contraction affects the perception of BC sound and the own voice is currently not clear.

Bone Conduction in Relation to Hearing Protection

People who are exposed to high-level sounds should protect the ears with hearing protection devices. In the extreme environments, the noise can exceed 150 dB SPL, and conventional hearing protection devices are no longer sufficient. Even if earplugs and earmuffs attenuate the AC pathway of sound to the cochlea, sound is reaching the cochlea by BC transmission. The head and body in a sound field is affected by the sound field, and BC sound is induced and transmitted to the cochlea. This sound field-induced BC sound limits the possible attenuation by conventional earmuffs and earplugs. According to Reinfeldt et al. [53], the BC transmission is 50–60 dB below the AC sensitivity at frequencies below 1 kHz, 40–50 dB at 2 kHz and 50–60 dB below the AC sensitivity at the higher frequencies. Consequently, to achieve more than 60 dB attenuation, the BC sound transmission needs to be attenuated as well. This can be accomplished by helmets or body covers.

Implications for Bone Conduction Hearing Aid Usage

Recent understanding of BC sound and sound transmission in the skull has indicated that the gain in sensitivity by stimulating close to the cochlea can overcome drawbacks of transcutaneous signal transmission for implantable BC hearing aids [54]. Also, for bilateral application of BC sound a position close to the cochlea results in greater interaural separation and would be beneficial for binaural processing abilities [38, 39]. However, when BC hearing aids are used with patients suffering from unilateral deafness, a positioning close to the cochlea does not improve the transcranial transmission, but does not decrease it either. It should be noted here that bilateral application of BC hearing aids does not only enable (reduced) binaural hearing, it also gives hearing from the non-hearing side (in a monaural fitting) and thereby removes the head-shadow effect – the primary reason for giving a BC hearing aid in unilateral deafness [55]. Consequently, giving a second BC hearing aid to a bilateral conductive-impaired patient provides greater benefit than giving a BC hearing aid to a unilateral deaf patient since no binaural processing is possible for the latter.

References

1 Ng M, Jackler R: Early history of tuning-fork tests. Am J Otolaryngol 1993;14:100–105.
2 Valentine M, Stark E: Bone conducted speech audiometry with normal-hearing and hearing-impaired children. J Aud Res 1977;17:105–108.
3 Purcell D, Kunov H, Madsen P, Cleghorn W: Distortion product otoacoustic emissions stimulated through bone conduction. Ear Hear 1998;19:362–370.
4 Beattie R: Normative Wave V latency-intensity functions using the EARTONE 3A insert earphone and the Radioear B-71 bone vibrator. Scand Audiol 1998;27:120–126.

5 Stenfelt S, Reinfeldt S: A model of the occlusion effect with bone-conducted stimulation. Int J Audiol 2007;46: 595–608.
6 International Organization for Standardization: Acoustics – reference zero for the calibration of audiometric equipment. 3. Reference equivalent threshold force levels for pure tones and bone vibrators. Geneva, International Organization for Standardization, 1994, ISO 389-3.
7 Popelka G, Telukuntla G, Puria S: Middle-ear function at high frequencies quantified with advanced bone-conduction measures. Hear Res 2010; 263:85–92.
8 Håkansson B: The balanced electromagnetic separation transducer: a new bone conduction transducer. J Acoust Soc Am 2003;113:818–825.
9 Weece R, Allen J: A method for calibration of bone driver transducers to measure the mastoid impedance. Hear Res 2010;263:216–223.
10 Richter U, Brinkmann K: Threshold of hearing by bone conduction. Scand Audiol 1981;10:235–237.
11 Minor LB: Superior canal dehiscence syndrome. Am J Otol 2000;21:9–19.
12 Stenfelt S, Håkansson B: Air versus bone conduction: an equal loudness investigation. Hear Res 2002;167:1–12.
13 von Békésy G: Zur theorie des hörens bei der schallaufnahme durch knochenleitung. Ann Physik 1932;13:111–136.
14 Khanna SM, Tonndorf J, Queller J: Mechanical parameters of hearing by bone conduction. J Acoust Soc Am 1976; 60:139–154.
15 Stenfelt S: Simultaneous cancellation of air and bone conduction tones at two frequencies: extension of the famous experiment by von Békésy. Hear Res 2007;225:105–116.
16 Stenfelt S, Puria S, Hato N, Goode RL: Basilar membrane and osseous spiral lamina motion in human cadavers with air and bone conduction stimuli. Hear Res 2003;181:131–143.
17 Mauldin L, Jerger J: Auditory brain stem evoked responses to bone-conducted signals. Arch Otolaryngol 1979;105: 656–661.
18 von Békésy G: Paradoxical direction of wave travel along the cochlear partition. J Acoust Soc Am 1955;27:137–145.
19 von Békésy G: Experiments in Hearing. New York, McGraw-Hill, 1960.
20 Tonndorf J: Bone conduction. Studies in experimental animals. Acta Otolaryngol 1966;(suppl 213):1–132.
21 Stenfelt S, Goode RL: Bone conducted sound: physiological and clinical aspects. Otol Neurotol 2005;26:1245–1261.
22 Stenfelt S, Wild T, Hato N, Goode RL: Factors contributing to bone conduction: the outer ear. J Acoust Soc Am 2003;113:902–912.
23 von Békésy G: Uber die Schallausbreitung bei Knochenleitung. Z Hals Nasen Ohrenheilk 1941;47:430–442.
24 Stenfelt S, Hato N, Goode RL: Factors contributing to bone conduction: the middle ear. J Acoust Soc Am 2002;111: 947–959.
25 Homma K, Du Y, Shimizu Y, Puria S: Ossicular resonance modes of the human middle ear for bone and air conduction. J Acoust Soc Am 2009;125: 968–979.
26 Hato N, Stenfelt S, Goode RL: Three-dimensional stapes footplate motion in human temporal bones. Audiol Neurootol 2003;8:140–152.
27 Carhart R: Effects of stapes fixation on bone-conduction response; in Ventry I, Chaiklin J, Dixon R (eds): Hearing Measurement: A book of Readings. New York, Appleton-Century-Crofts, 1971, pp 116–129.
28 Huizing EH: Bone conduction – the influence of the middle ear. Acta Otolaryngol 1960;suppl 155:1–99.
29 Stenfelt S: Middle ear ossicles motion at hearing thresholds with air conduction and bone conduction stimulation. J Acoust Soc Am 2006;119:2848–2858.
30 Ranke O, Keidel W, Weschke H: Das Hören beim Verschluss des runden Fensters. Zeit Laryngol 1952;31:467–475.
31 Kucuk B, Abe K, Ushiki T: Microstructures of the bony modiolus in the human cochlea: scanning electron microscopic study. J Electron Microsc 1991;40:193–197.
32 Songer J, Rosowski J: A superior semicircular canal dehiscence-induced air-bone gap in chinchilla. Hear Res 2010;269: 70–80.
33 Sohmer H, Freeman S, Geal-Dor M, Adelman C, Savion I: Bone conduction experiments in humans – a fluid pathway from bone to ear. Hear Res 2000; 146:81–88.
34 Yoshida M, Uemura T: Transmission of cerebrospinal fluid pressure changes to the inner ear and its effect on cochlear microphonics. Eur Arch Otorhinolaryngol 1991;248:139–143.
35 Håkansson B, Brandt A, Carlsson P, Tjellström A: Resonance frequency of the human skull in vivo. J Acoust Soc Am 1994;95:1474–1481.
36 Håkansson B, Carlsson P, Brandt A, Stenfelt S: Linearity of sound transmission through the human skull in vivo. J Acoust Soc Am 1996;99:2239–2243.
37 Stenfelt S, Håkansson B, Tjellström A: Vibration characteristics of bone conducted sound in vitro. J Acoust Soc Am 2000;107:422–431.
38 Stenfelt S, Goode RL: Transmission properties of bone conducted sound: measurements in cadaver heads. J Acoust Soc Am 2005;118:2373–2391.
39 Eeg-Olofsson M, Stenfelt S, Granström G: Implications for contralateral bone conducted transmission as measured by cochlear vibrations. Otol Neurotol 2010, Epub ahead of print.
40 Eeg-Olofsson M, Stenfelt S, Tjellström A, Granström G: Transmission of bone-conducted sound in the human skull measured by cochlear vibrations. Int J Audiol 2008;47:761–769.
41 Stenfelt S, Håkansson B: Sensitivity to bone-conducted sound: excitation of the mastoid vs the teeth. Scand Audiol 1999; 28:190–198.
42 Snik AF, Mylanus EAM, Proops DW, Wolfaardt JF, Hodgetts WE, Somers T, Niparko JK, Wazen JJ, Sterkers O, Cremers CWRJ, Tjellström A: Consensus statements on the Baha system: where do we stand at present? Ann Otol Rhinol Laryngol 2005;114(suppl 195):1–12.
43 Nolan M, Lyon DJ: Transcranial attenuation in bone conduction audiometry. J Laryngol Otol 1981;95:597–608.
44 Privin C, Stenfelt S, Granström G, Tjellström A, Håkansson B: Bilateral bone-anchored hearing aids (Bahas): an audiometric evaluation. Laryngoscope 2004;114:77–84.
45 Bosman A, Snik A, van der Pouw C, Mylanus E, Cramers C: Audiometric evaluation of bilaterally fitted bone-anchored hearing aids. Audiology 2001;40:158–167.
46 Rowan D, Gray M: Lateralization of high-frequency pure tones with interaural phase difference and bone conduction. Int J Audiol 2008;47:404–411.

47 MacDonald J, Henry P, Letowski T: Spatial audio through a bone conduction interface. Int J Audiol 2006;45:595–599.
48 von Békésy G: The structure of the middle ear and the hearing of one's own voice by bone conduction. J Acoust Soc Am 1949;21:217–232.
49 Pörschmann C: Influences of bone conduction and air conduction on the sound of one's own voice. Acustica 2000; 86:1038–1045.
50 Reinfeldt S, Ostli P, Håkansson B, Stenfelt S: Hearing one's own voice during phoneme vocalization – transmission by air and bone conduction. J Acoust Soc Am 2010;128:751–762.
51 Bárány E: A contribution to the physiology of bone conduction. Acta Otolaryngol 1938;(suppl 26):1–223.
52 Borg E, Zakrisson J: The activity of the stapedius muscle in man during vocalization. Acta Otolaryngol 1975;79: 325–333.
53 Reinfeldt S, Stenfelt S, Good T, Håkansson B: Examination of bone-conducted transmission from sound field excitation measured by thresholds, ear-canal sound pressure, and skull vibrations. J Acoust Soc Am 2007;121: 1576–1587.
54 Håkansson B, Reinfeldt S, Eeg-Olofsson M, Ostli P, Taghavi H, Adler J, Gabrielsson J, Stenfelt S, Granström G: A novel bone conduction implant (BCI): engineering aspects and pre-clinical studies. Int J Audiol 2010;49:203–215.
55 Stenfelt S: Bilateral fitting of Bahas and Baha fitted in unilateral deaf persons: acoustical aspects. Int J Audiol 2005;44: 178–189.

Stefan Stenfelt
Department of Clinical and Experimental Medicine
Technical Audiology, Linköping University
SE–58185 Linköping (Sweden)
Tel. +46 10 1032856, E-Mail stefan.stenfelt@liu.se

Kompis M, Caversaccio M-D (eds): Implantable Bone Conduction Hearing Aids.
Adv Otorhinolaryngol. Basel, Karger, 2011, vol 71, pp 22–31

An Overview of Different Systems: The Bone-Anchored Hearing Aid

Catharina A.J. Dun · Hubert T. Faber · Maarten J.F. de Wolf · Cor W.R.J. Cremers · Myrthe K.S. Hol

Department of Otorhinolaryngology, Donders Institute for Brain, Cognition and Behaviour, Radboud University Nijmegen Medical Centre, Nijmegen, The Netherlands

Abstract

In the past 30 years, a large amount of clinical and audiological research on bone conduction hearing devices has been performed. In this review, we give a brief history of the developments in indications, surgical techniques and sound processors with respect to implantable bone conduction devices like the bone-anchored hearing aid or Baha. Starting with the use of Baha in patients with bilateral conductive or mixed hearing loss (HL), the indications for such devices have been extended to patients with unilateral HL, children and moderate mentally retarded patients. Bilateral fitting has been shown to be beneficial in restoring binaural hearing in patients with bilateral acquired or congenital conductive HL. In addition, the surgical techniques used to implant the titanium fixture for Baha application have been modified and further developed to reach two main goals: (a) optimal osseointegration, and (b) preparation of the implant site to minimize the occurrence of soft tissue reactions. Currently, the most used techniques are the pedicled skin flap, dermatome and linear incision techniques. Several generations of the Baha® sound processor have been developed by Cochlear™ to provide sufficient amplification in different hearing situations. Improvements in sound quality, aesthetics and handling have been major points of interest. The Baha sound processors most often used today are the Baha® Divino, the Baha® Intenso and the Baha® Cordelle. Recently, the more flexible Baha® BP100 sound processor was launched.

Introduction

In 1984, the bone-anchored hearing aid (Baha), which was developed by Håkansson, Tjellström and coworkers in Gothenburg, Sweden, became commercially available [1]. Currently, the Baha is a well-established device for hearing rehabilitation for conductive hearing loss (HL), and over 250 papers have been published worldwide on this hearing device. In June 1988, the first 3 Nijmegen patients were fitted with a Baha device [2], setting off more than 20 years of clinical and audiological research and resulting in more than 50 publications in various Baha-related fields. In this review, we give an overview of current knowledge about the Baha in general, with special attention given to research performed over the past several years in our clinic.

Physiology of Bone Conduction

The physiological concept behind the bone conduction (BC) pathway is still not entirely understood. Tonndorf [3] described, from studies primarily in cats, several modes stimulating the basilar membrane during BC excitation. The significance of the different modes depends on the frequency. For humans at hearing frequencies, the most important way in which the basilar membrane is stimulated seems to be the effect of fluid inertia within the cochlear [4, 5]. In short, BC sound is made up of vibrations transmitted through the skull to the cochlea. This then causes the fluids in the cochlea to vibrate as well. As these fluids are incompressible in principle, they will vibrate as a whole and in phase with the bone. However, the cochlea has two mobile windows, the oval and the round window. Therefore, inertia of the inner ear fluids will result in longitudinal fluid waves traveling from one window to the other, which causes the basilar membrane to vibrate.

Von Békésy [6] showed that the basilar membrane responds equally to both air-conducted (AC) and BC sound. To distinguish between AC and BC stimulation at the basilar membrane level is not possible. However, the BC route towards the basilar membrane is energywise less efficient than the air conduction route. Therefore, BC hearing aids are primarily used for HL where air conduction hearing aids are contraindicated.

Description of the Baha System

The Baha® is a semi-implantable percutaneous BC hearing device coupled to the skull by an osseointegrated titanium fixture (fig. 1). The titanium fixture used is a standard Brånemark type of implant with an as-machined surface, developed by Cochlear™ Bone Anchored Solutions, Gothenburg, Sweden. Recently, as there have been substantial developments of titanium fixtures for the dental industry, a new Baha® BI300 implant has been designed to improve stability and to enhance osseointegration. The new Baha BI300 implant features a wider diameter (4.5 mm compared to 3.75 mm for the standard implant), small sized threads at the implant neck, and a moderately rough TiOblast™ surface on the intraosseous portion of the implant. Figure 2 illustrates the standard titanium implant and the new BI300 implant (fig. 2). A skin-penetrating abutment is attached to the implant to facilitate coupling of the Baha sound processor. Compared to the standard abutment, the BI300 abutment is a concave-shaped abutment. The direct coupling for the mechanical vibrations to the skull provides effective sound transmission of around 5–15 dB higher than the transcutaneous coupling of conventional BC devices [7]. Because the Baha sound processor is coupled directly to the skull without interference from intermediate tissue, some drawbacks of conventional transcutaneous BC devices are avoided. These drawbacks include pressure of the transducer mounted on a spring or in the sidepiece of spectacles against the temporal skin, which can result in headaches or skin reactions and insufficient pressure, which reduces the

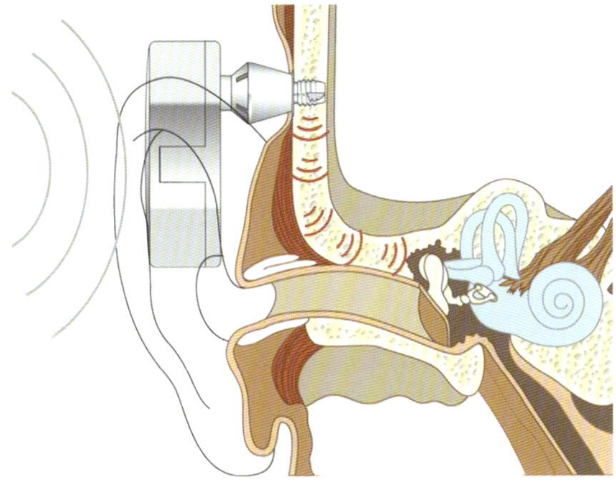

Fig. 1. Illustration of the Baha as a semi-implantable percutaneous BC hearing device coupled to the skull by an osseointegrated titanium fixture.

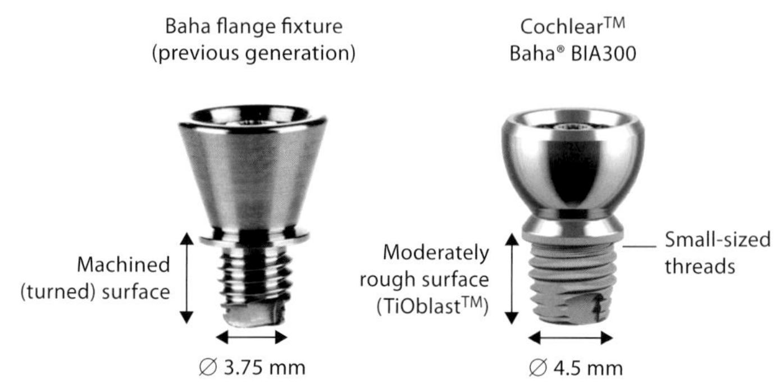

Fig. 2. Illustration of the standard titanium implant (left) and the new BI300 titanium implant (right).

gain of the device. Furthermore, when the classical bone conductor is used with a headband, mostly, the positioning of the microphone and vibrational transducer are contralaterally on the skull, resulting in unnatural listening conditions. The same drawbacks apply to conventional BC devices with the amplifier worn on the body. On the other hand, the disadvantages of percutaneous implants include loss of osseointegration and skin reactions around the implant.

Indications

Bilateral Mixed or Conductive Hearing Loss (Acquired/Congenital)
The Baha system is typically beneficial in patients with bilateral mixed or conductive HL who cannot be fitted with conventional acoustic hearing aids (behind the ear or in the ear), including those with chronic otitis and those with congenital aural atresia [8–10]. In patients for whom reconstructive surgery is no longer considered a feasible option and for whom a conventional BC hearing aid has proven to be inadequate, the Baha has been shown to be of great benefit [11–16].

Whereas most bilateral hearing-impaired patients with sensorineural HL, using acoustic hearing aids prefer binaural amplification over monaural amplification, binaural use of the Baha in bilaterally impaired patients is not yet widely applied.

There are several well-documented advantages of binaural hearing: (a) hearing sensitivity and speech recognition are improved due to bilateral summation when inputs received by the two cochleae are added together [17, 18], (b) speech recognition is improved in noisy situations with spatially separated speech and noise sources [19], and (c) directional hearing will be enabled in the horizontal plane. It has been reported that bilateral Baha use in adults has both significant subjective and objective benefits [14, 20].

Unilateral Conductive Hearing Loss
Unilateral conductive HL (UCHL) in patients with a contralateral normal hearing ear may involve the typical problems associated with unilateral hearing (i.e. poor sound localization abilities and poor speech recognition performance in noise). Agterberg et al. [21] reported on sound localization in patients with acquired UCHL fitted with a BC device (BCD) on their impaired side. Using varied several stimulus characteristics, they demonstrated that BCD users with acquired UCHL were able to localize sounds on the basis of restored binaural hearing; see also the chapter by Agterberg et al. [this vol.]. However,

some UCHL patients show fairly good directional hearing abilities in an unaided monaural condition [22, 23].

Single-Sided Deafness
In patients with unilateral sensorineural deafness, a Baha positioned near the deaf ear works as a transcranial CROS (contralateral routing of signal). Sounds received by the Baha system are transmitted to the functional contralateral cochlea via BC. In principle, this will not result in stereophonic hearing, but the negative effects of acoustic head shadow (poor understanding of a person who is talking on the deaf side of the patient) might be decreased [24, 25]. Before implantation, a trial should be arranged with a Baha device on a steel headband placed on the mastoid of the deaf ear [26]. The degree of success depends on the motivation of the patient and the listening demands imposed by their lifestyle and working environment. In the literature, it is reported that 25–30% of the patients apply for implantation of the Baha® system after trial on a headband [24, 27].

Baha Use in Children
In part, Baha application in children addresses different issues than in adults. Children are known to have more immature and thinner bone. When implanted, they have a higher risk of soft tissue overgrowth, and, compared to adults, more implants are lost within the first year after implantation [28]. Furthermore, cleaning problems have been reported, especially among adolescents [29, 30]. A considerable number of the children scheduled for implantation have major congenital (syndromal) malformations of the ear, sometimes combined with skull deformities, making surgery more challenging [31–34]. For Baha surgery in children, there are additional considerations and precautions, including (a) at what age is implantation possible, (b) what should be the minimal thickness of the skull bone, (c) what is the best implant position, (d) is there a need to place a second sleeping fixture, and (e) what can be done to prevent postsurgery soft tissue reactions. It is of the utmost importance that children with bilateral conductive HL be rehabilitated at the earliest age possible as early and consistent stimulation is critical for optimal development of speech and language [35].

For children who are too young to be fitted with a Baha percutaneously, and to overcome the risks associated with Baha surgery in specific syndromal cases, a conventional transcutaneous bone conductor can be used or the more recently introduced Baha® Softband (Cochlear Bone-Anchored Solutions). This Baha Softband comprises the Baha sound processor connected to a soft elastic headband. Aided sound field thresholds with the Baha Softband are almost equivalent to those obtained with a transcutaneous conventional BC hearing aid [36]. Speech and language development are greatly facilitated by the early use of bone-conductors like the Baha Softband [37], and currently, the Baha Softband is generally accepted as the treatment for children under 3 years of age.

Lieu [38] and Lieu et al. [39] found that several children with unilateral HL demonstrate increased rates of school year failure and that they needed additional educational assistance. The Paediatric Workgroup on Hearing Aid Amplification [40] summarized the literature and stated that in children with unilateral conductive or sensorineural HL, amplification should be considered on a case-by-case basis, centered on the child's audiometric data, development, and communication needs.

Baha Use in Patients with Moderate Mental Retardation
Initially, potential Baha patients with mental retardation were excluded from treatment due to doubts concerning care for the percutaneous implant and surrounding skin. Recently, however, patients with moderate mental retardation and conductive or mixed HL have received Baha treatment. Use of the Baha in this specific patient

group has been shown to be beneficial, improving both listening and learning capabilities [41–43]. Following these results, use of the Baha has also been extended as a valuable treatment option for this special patient group.

Baha Surgery

Goals of Surgery

Independent of the surgical technique used, there are two major goals of Baha surgery: placement of an implant capable of optimal osseointegration and preparation of an implant site that minimizes the occurrence of future soft tissue reactions surrounding the implant. For adequate osseointegration, trauma to the surrounding bone should be minimized. The actual placement (drilling and placing) of the implant is mostly done using the technique reported by Tjellström [44]. Subcutaneous tissue reduction is carried out to reduce soft tissue movement and the subsequent development of scar tissue and infection around the implant. In addition, hair follicles surrounding the implant should be removed to avoid skin irritation and accumulation of debris. If all of these precautions are taken into consideration and therapy-resistant skin reactions still occur, recent studies have shown that changing to a larger 8.5-mm abutment can be beneficial [45–47]. A recent study by Faber et al. [48] showed that implant location was not correlated with the frequency and severity of skin reactions around the abutment in 248 randomly selected Baha patients.

Handling Soft Tissue (Surgical Techniques)

The surgical techniques used to handle soft tissue vary among surgeons. Initially, a free retroauricular skin graft was used, which later became a local pedicled skin flap predominantly [33, 49, 50]. To standardize the surgical flap technique, a special dermatome was developed to create a hair free, thin, skin flap [49, 51]. An alternative surgical technique, using a linear incision, has been developed at the Radboud University Nijmegen Medical [52–54]. Both the dermatome technique and linear incision technique provide safe alternatives in Baha surgery and are recommended in the Baha® Surgery Guide (Cochlear) [55].

Loading Time

Another point of interest in previous studies has been osseointegration of the titanium implant. Osseointegration of the implant is key to the success of the Baha implant before loading the implant with the Baha sound device. In 2005, Snik et al. [26] published a consensus report by experts in the field recommending a loading time of between 4 and 6 weeks in adults and at least 3 months in children under 10 years of age. In accordance with this report, the current protocol for Baha surgery (Cochlear) includes 6 weeks of unloaded healing to allow for sufficient osseointegration and stability of the implant in adults [55]. In children with bone thickness of 3–4 mm, two-stage surgery is recommended and the Baha sound processor can be attached as soon as wound healing has occurred after the second stage. Longer healing time before loading should still be used in adults being irradiated on the skull bone, in adults with bony disorders and when soft bone is observed during initial fixture implantation.

Development of Different Generations of the Baha Sound Processors

Since the introduction, several Baha sound processors have been developed. The first commercially available device was the HC 200, released in 1987. Since this release, updates have been made to approach more specific hearing needs. Also the aesthetical aspects were taken into consideration in these updates, the size of the processor was minimized and different colors were made available. Nowadays, there are four types of Baha sound processors (Cochlear) commercially available: the Baha® Divino, the Baha®

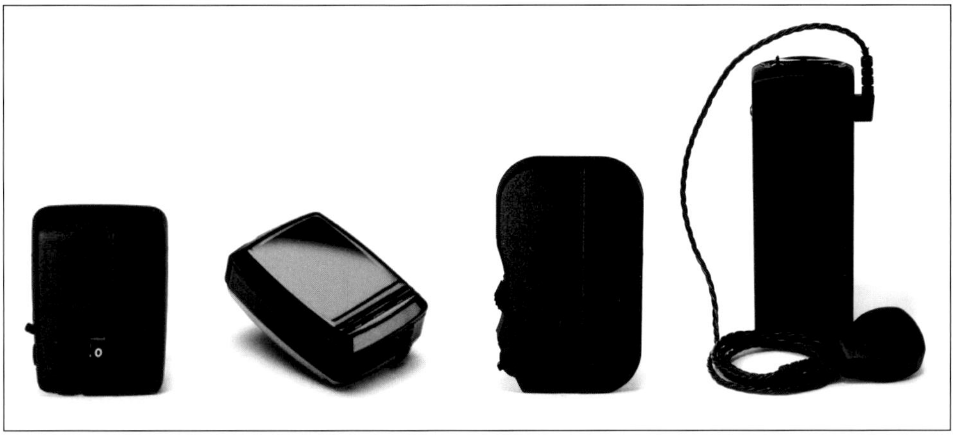

Fig. 3. Available Baha sound processors (left to right): Baha Divino, new Baha BP100, Baha Intenso and Baha Cordelle with bodyworn receiver (not actual sizes).

BP100, the Baha® Intenso and the Baha® Cordelle (fig. 3). The Divino, Intenso and the BP100 are behind-the-ear devices containing microphone, amplifier and vibration transducer in one casing. The Baha Cordelle consists of a separate ear level vibration transducer connected to a bodyworn microphone and amplifier. In 1993, this Baha Cordelle was designed out from preceding processors such as the HC Superbass as an even more powerful successor [56]. The Baha Divino was launched in 2005. In contrast to its predecessor, the Baha Compact, this device features a digital sound processor and a directional microphone. Sound-field thresholds and speech tests in quiet did not reveal any statistically significant advantage (or disadvantage) of the Baha Divino when compared to the Baha Compact [57]. However, speech understanding in noise presented at the rear was reported to be better with the Baha Divino, an effect assigned to the directional microphone noise-reduction system. The Baha Intenso, launched in 2007, bridges the gap between the Baha Divino and the Baha Cordelle. Of the ear-level Baha (i.e. Cordelle not included), the Baha Intenso provides the most gain and the highest maximum output.

To determine the fitting range of three most used types of Baha devices, speech recognition data on three groups of Baha users were obtained from the Nijmegen database. Figure 4 presents the (monaural) individual aided phoneme scores in quiet at 65 dB SPL (sound pressure level; PS65) from 90 Baha Compact (predecessor Divino) users, 23 Baha Intenso users and 25 Baha Cordelle users (fig. 4). All patients had conductive HL or mixed HL, with a sensorineural HL component of up to 70 dB HL. PS65 was presented as function of the mean sensorineural HL component. Nonlinear regression curves of the second order were fitted through the individual data and are also presented. Using these lines, it was concluded that for a sensorineural HL component exceeding approximately 25 dB, scores were better with the stronger Baha Intenso than with the Compact. At this threshold, the PS65 line of the Baha Compact was 10% lower (arbitrary choice) than that of the Baha Intenso, and the discrepancy continued to increase with increasing sensorineural HL component. Therefore, assuming that the speech tests in quiet of the Baha Compact and its successor Baha Divino are equally effective, it can

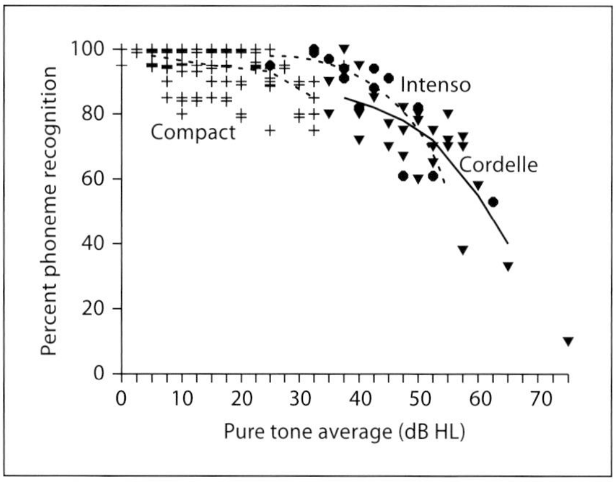

Fig. 4. (Monaural) individual aided phoneme scores in quiet at 65 dB SPL (PS65) from three groups of Baha users presented as function of their mean sensorineural hearing loss. The three lines are best-fitted nonlinear regression lines.

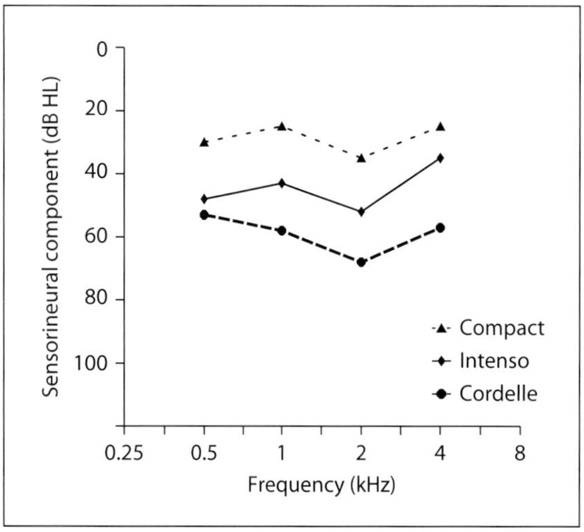

Fig. 5. Audiological application range for three types of Baha devices. The Baha Divino and also the Baha BP100 are expected to have application ranges comparable to their predecessor the Baha Compact.

be established that the Baha Divino is a good choice for patients with a mild sensorineural HL component of up to 25 dB HL.

In a similar way, the upper limit of application for the Baha Intenso was set at 50 dB HL. At this threshold, the PS65 with a Baha Cordelle was likely to be at least 10% higher than with the Baha Intenso. The Baha Intenso is a good choice for patients with an average sensorineural HL component of between 30 and 50 dB HL (fig. 4) [58].

Bosman et al. [59] assessed the upper level fitting range of the Baha Cordelle in patients with severe to profound mixed HL. To reach a 50% score at 65 dB, the upper limit of the fitting range as expressed in BC thresholds was set to 50, 55, 65, 60 dB HL at 500, 1,000, 2,000 and 4,000 Hz, respectively. If the gain is insufficient for a particular patient, the next amplification option is the application of a cochlear implant. From a more recent study by Verhaegen et al. [60] it was concluded that a CI takes preference over a Baha device in patients with mixed HL when the mean sensorineural HL component is 65–70 dB or higher or when the PS65 with the Baha Cordelle is less than about 40%.

With the aid of information on the gain-frequency characteristics of Baha, as measured in patients, the straightforward application limits can be shaped into frequencies. The gain-frequency relations have been described in a group of patients using the Baha Intenso and Baha Cordelle [58, 59]. Using these frequency-gain data as input and the National Acoustics Laboratory-Non-Linear (NAL-N-L) rule backwards, frequency-specific hearing thresholds can be obtained instead of a mean hearing threshold. The NAL-N-L rule is a well-validated prescription method that prescribes desired gain based on hearing thresholds [61, 62]. Figure 4 shows the final result for change from Compact to Intenso and from Intenso to Cordelle (fig. 5). The figure can be used to choose the best Baha option for Baha candidates. The Baha Compact is not available anymore, and application data can be used for its successors, the Baha Divino and the Baha BP100.

Towards the end of 2009, a new Baha sound processor was launched, the Baha BP100. The

BP100 is considered to be applicable in individuals with bone conduction thresholds up to 35 dB. This device makes use of full digital processing. With this device, sound is analyzed across 12 channels. It has several automatic systems that operate on the incoming sound signal such as adaptive amplification and automatic noise reduction. Another special feature is that hearing thresholds can be measured directly by stimulation by pure tones generated by the BP100 sound processor such that the gain can be adapted individually and frequency specific [63]. A first clinical evaluation showed that compared with the Baha Divino, speech understanding in noise was on average 2.6 dB better with the Baha BP100 [64]. In this evaluation, the sound quality of the BP100, assessed by a patient's questionnaire, was reported to be better compared to the Divino. Company-independent effectivity studies of the Baha BP 100 have not yet been published and should be awaited for.

Recently, alternative implantable bone-conduction devices produced by other companies entered the field. Oticon Medical received clearance from the US Food and Drug Administration to market their percutaneous Ponto® system; see also the chapter by Westerkull [this vol.]. In 2010, the Sophono, Inc., and Otomag GmbH companies have teamed together to pioneer the development of a non-percutaneous implantable BC device, called the Otomag Alpha® [65]; see also the chapter by Siegert [this vol.].

References

1 Hakansson B, Tjellström A, Rosenhall U, Carlsson P: The bone-anchored hearing aid. Principal design and a psychoacoustical evaluation. Acta Otolaryngol 1985; 100:229–239.
2 Cremers CWRJ, Snik AFM, Beynon AJ: A hearing aid anchored in the cranial bone for amplification of bone conduction. Ned Tijdschr Geneeskd 1991;135: 468–471.
3 Tonndorf J: Animal experiments in bone conduction: clinical conclusions. Trans Am Otol Soc 1964;52:22–43.
4 Stenfelt S, Goode RL: Transmission properties of bone conducted sound: measurements in cadaver heads. J Acoust Soc Am 2005;118:2373–2391.
5 Stenfelt S, Goode RL: Bone-conducted sound: physiological and clinical aspects. Otol Neurotol 2005;26:1245–1261.
6 von Békésy G: Current status of theories of hearing. Science 1956;123:779–783.
7 Stenfelt SP, Hakansson BE: A miniaturized artificial mastoid using a skull simulator. Scand Audiol 1998;27:67–76.
8 Mylanus EAM, Snik AFM, Cremers CWRJ: Patients' opinions of bone-anchored vs conventional hearing aids. Arch Otolaryngol Head Neck Surg 1995; 121:421–425.
9 Mylanus EAM, van der Pouw CTM, Snik AFM, Cremers CWRJ: Intraindividual comparison of the bone-anchored hearing aid and air-conduction hearing aids. Arch Otolaryngol Head Neck Surg 1998;124:271–276.
10 Hol MKS, Snik AFM, Mylanus EAM, Cremers CWRJ: Long-term results of bone-anchored hearing aid recipients who had previously used air-conduction hearing aids. Arch Otolaryngol Head Neck Surg 2005;131:321–325.
11 Wazen JJ, Caruso M, Tjellström A: Long-term results with the titanium bone-anchored hearing aid: the U.S. experience. Am J Otol 1998;19:737–741.
12 Arunachalam PS, Kilby D, Meikle D, Davison T, Johnson IJ: Bone-anchored hearing aid quality of life assessed by Glasgow Benefit Inventory. Laryngoscope 2001;111:1260–1263.
13 Cooper HR, Burrell SP, Powell RH, Proops DW, Bickerton JA: The Birmingham bone anchored hearing aid programme: referrals, selection, rehabilitation, philosophy and adult results. J Laryngol Otol 1996;21(suppl): 13–20.
14 Dutt SN, McDermott AL, Burrell SP, Cooper HR, Reid AP, Proops DW: Patient satisfaction with bilateral bone-anchored hearing aids: the Birmingham experience. J Laryngol Otol Suppl 2002; 116:37–46.
15 Dutt SN, McDermott AL, Jelbert A, Reid AP, Proops DW: The Glasgow benefit inventory in the evaluation of patient satisfaction with the bone-anchored hearing aid: quality of life issues. J Laryngol Otol Suppl 2002;116:7–14.
16 Hol MKS, Spath MA, Krabbe PFM, van der Pouw CTM, Snik AFM, Cremers CWRJ, Mylanus EAM: The bone-anchored hearing aid: quality-of-life assessment. Arch Otolaryngol Head Neck Surg 2004;130:394–399.
17 Snik AFM, Beynon AJ, Mylanus EAM, van der Pouw CTM, Cremers CWRJ: Binaural application of the bone-anchored hearing aid. Ann Otol Rhinol Laryngol 1998;107:187–193.
18 van der Pouw CTM, Snik AFM, Cremers CWRJ: Audiometric results of bilateral bone-anchored hearing aid application in patients with bilateral congenital aural atresia. Laryngoscope 1998;108: 548–553.

19 Bosman AJ, Snik AFM, van der Pouw CTM, Mylanus EAM, Cremers CWRJ: Audiometric evaluation of bilaterally fitted bone-anchored hearing aids. Audiology 2001;40:158–167.
20 Dutt SN, McDermott AL, Burrell SP, Cooper HR, Reid AP, Proops DW: Speech intelligibility with bilateral bone-anchored hearing aids: the Birmingham experience. J Laryngol Otol Suppl 2002; 28:47–51.
21 Agterberg MJ, Snik AFM, Hol MKS, van Esch TE, Cremers CWRJ, Van Wanrooij MM, Van Opstal AJ: Improved horizontal directional hearing in bone conduction device users with acquired unilateral conductive hearing loss. J Assoc Res Otolaryngol 2010, Epub ahead of print.
22 Priwin C, Jonsson R, Hultcrantz M, Granström G: BAHA in children and adolescents with unilateral or bilateral conductive hearing loss: a study of outcome. Int J Pediatr Otorhinolaryngol 2007;71:135–145.
23 Snik AFM, Mylanus EAM, Cremers CWRJ: The bone-anchored hearing aid in patients with a unilateral air-bone gap. Otol Neurotol 2002;23:61–66.
24 Hol MKS, Bosman AJ, Snik AFM, Mylanus EAM, Cremers CWRJ: Bone-anchored hearing aid in unilateral inner ear deafness: a study of 20 patients. Audiol Neurootol 2004;9:274–281.
25 Niparko JK, Cox KM, Lustig LR: Comparison of the bone anchored hearing aid implantable hearing device with contralateral routing of offside signal amplification in the rehabilitation of unilateral deafness. Otol Neurotol 2003;24:73–78.
26 Snik AFM, Mylanus EAM, Proops DW, Wolfaardt JF, Hodgetts WE, Somers T, et al: Consensus statements on the BAHA system: where do we stand at present? Ann Otol Rhinol Laryngol 2005;195(suppl):2–12.
27 Andersen HT, Schroder SA, Bonding P: Unilateral deafness after acoustic neuroma surgery: subjective hearing handicap and the effect of the bone-anchored hearing aid. Otol Neurotol 2006;27: 809–814.
28 De Wolf MJF, Hol MKS, Huygen PL, Mylanus EAM, Cremers CWRJ: Nijmegen results with application of a bone-anchored hearing aid in children: simplified surgical technique. Ann Otol Rhinol Laryngol 2008;117:805–814.
29 Granström G: Osseointegrated implants in children. Acta Otolaryngol Suppl 2000;543:118–121.
30 Lloyd S, Almeyda J, Sirimanna KS, Albert DM, Bailey CM: Updated surgical experience with bone-anchored hearing aids in children. J Laryngol Otol 2007;121:826–831.
31 Granström G, Bergström K, Odersjo M, Tjellström A: Osseointegrated implants in children: experience from our first 100 patients. Otolaryngol Head Neck Surg 2001;125:85–92.
32 McDermott AL, Williams J, Kuo M, Reid A, Proops D: The Birmingham Pediatric Bone-Anchored Hearing Aid Program: a 15-year experience. Otol Neurotol 2009;30:178–183.
33 Tjellström A, Hakansson B, Granström G: Bone-anchored hearing aids: current status in adults and children. Otolaryngol Clin North Am 2001;34: 337–364.
34 Zeitoun H, De R, Thompson SD, Proops DW: Osseointegrated implants in the management of childhood ear abnormalities: with particular emphasis on complications. J Laryngol Otol 2002;116: 87–91.
35 Yoshinaga-Itano C: Early intervention after universal neonatal hearing screening: impact on outcomes. Ment Retard Dev Disabil Res Rev 2003;9:252–266.
36 Hol MKS, Cremers CWRJ, Coppens-Schellekens W, Snik AFM: The BAHA Softband. A new treatment for young children with bilateral congenital aural atresia. Int J Pediatr Otorhinolaryngol 2005;69:973–980.
37 Verhagen CV, Hol MKS, Coppens-Schellekens W, Snik AFM, Cremers CWRJ: The Baha Softband. A new treatment for young children with bilateral congenital aural atresia. Int J Pediatr Otorhinolaryngol 2008;72:1455–1459.
38 Lieu JE: Speech-language and educational consequences of unilateral hearing loss in children. Arch Otolaryngol Head Neck Surg 2004;130:524–530.
39 Lieu JE, Tye-Murray N, Karzon RK, Piccirillo JF: Unilateral hearing loss is associated with worse speech-language scores in children. Pediatrics 2010;125: e1348–e1355.
40 Bess FH, Chase PA, Gravel JS: Position statement on amplification for infants and children with hearing loss; in Seewald RC (ed): A Sound Foundation through Early Amplification. London, Ontario, Canada, 2010, pp 253–262.
41 Kunst SJW, Hol MKS, Cremers CWRJ, Mylanus EAM: Bone-anchored hearing aid in patients with moderate mental retardation: impact and benefit assessment. Otol Neurotol 2007;28:793–797.
42 McDermott AL, Williams J, Kuo MJ, Reid AP, Proops DW: The role of bone anchored hearing aids in children with Down syndrome. Int J Pediatr Otorhinolaryngol 2008;72:751–757.
43 Kunst SJW, Hol MKS, Snik AFM, Mylanus EAM, Cremers CWRJ: Rehabilitation of patients with conductive hearing loss and moderate mental retardation by means of a bone-anchored hearing aid. Otol Neurotol 2006;27:653–658.
44 Tjellström A: Osseointegrated systems and their application in the head and neck. Adv Otolaryngol Head Neck Surg 1989;3:39–70.
45 Doshi J, McDermott AL, Reid A, Proops D: The 8.5mm abutment in children: the Birmingham Bone-Anchored Hearing Aid Program experience. Otol Neurotol 2010;31:612–614.
46 Dun CAJ, Hol MKS, Mylanus EAM, Cremers CWRJ: Fitting of an 8.5mm abutment for bone-anchored hearing aids; indications and post-intervention course, submitted.
47 Monksfield P, Ho EC, Reid A, Proops D: Experience with the longer (8.5 mm) abutment for Bone-Anchored Hearing Aid. Otol Neurotol 2009;30:274–276.
48 Faber HT, De Wolf MJF, de Rooy JW, Hol MKS, Cremers CWRJ, Mylanus EAM: Bone-anchored hearing aid implant location in relation to skin reactions. Arch Otolaryngol Head Neck Surg 2009;135:742–747.
49 Tjellström A, Granström G: How we do it: frequency of skin necrosis after BAHA surgery. Clin Otolaryngol 2006;31: 216–220.
50 Proops DW: The Birmingham bone anchored hearing aid programme: surgical methods and complications. J Laryngol Otol Suppl 1996;21:7–12.
51 Stalfors J, Tjellström A: Skin reactions after BAHA surgery: a comparison between the U-graft technique and the BAHA dermatome. Otol Neurotol 2008; 29:1109–1114.
52 van der Pouw CTM, Mylanus EAM, Cremers CWRJ: Percutaneous implants in the temporal bone for securing a bone conductor: surgical methods and results. Ann Otol Rhinol Laryngol 1999;108: 532–536.

53 Mylanus EAM, Beynon AJ, Snik AFM, Cremers CWRJ: Percutaneous titanium implantation in the skull for the bone-anchored hearing aid. J Invest Surg 1994; 7:327–332.
54 De Wolf MJF, Hol MKS, Huygen PL, Mylanus EAM, Cremers CWRJ: Clinical outcome of the simplified surgical technique for BAHA implantation. Otol Neurotol 2008;29:1100–1108.
55 Cochlear Bone Anchored Solutions AB: Surgery Guide. Gothenburg, Cochlear Bone Anchored Solutions, 2010.
56 van der Pouw CTM, Carlsson P, Cremers CWRJ, Snik AFM: A new more powerful bone-anchored hearing aid: first results. Scand Audiol 1998;27:179–182.
57 Kompis M, Krebs M, Hausler R: Speech understanding in quiet and in noise with the bone-anchored hearing aids Baha Compact and Baha Divino. Acta Otolaryngol 2007;127:829–835.
58 Bosman AJ, Snik AFM, Mylanus EAM, Cremers CWRJ: Fitting range of the BAHA Intenso. Int J Audiol 2009;48: 346–352.
59 Bosman AJM, Snik AFM, Mylanus EAM, Cremers CWRJ: Fitting range of the BAHA Cordelle. Int J Audiol 2006;45: 429–437.
60 Verhaegen VJ, Mulder JJ, Mylanus EAM, Cremers CWRJ, Snik AFM: Profound mixed hearing loss: bone-anchored hearing aid system or cochlear implant? Ann Otol Rhinol Laryngol 2009;118: 693–697.
61 Dillon H, Storey L: The National Acoustic Laboratories' procedure for selecting the saturation sound pressure level of hearing aids: theoretical derivation. Ear Hear 1998;19:255–266.
62 Verhaegen VJ, Mylanus EA, Cremers CW, Snik AF: Audiological application criteria for implantable hearing aid devices: a clinical experience at the Nijmegen ORL clinic. Laryngoscope 2008;118:1645–1649.
63 Flynn MC, Hillbratt M: BC Direct – facilitating an individualized and accurate fitting of a Baha sound processor. Gothenburg, Cochlear Bone Anchored Solutions, E81512, 2009.
64 Flynn MC, Sadeghi A, Halvarsson G: Results of the first clinical evaluation of the Cochlear™ Baha® BP100. Gothenburg, Cochlear Bone Anchored Solutions, E81511, 2009.
65 Siegert R: Magnetic coupling of partially implantable bone conduction hearing aids without open implants. Laryngorhinootologie 2010;89:346–351.

Myrthe K.S. Hol
Department of Otorhinolaryngology, Radboud University Nijmegen Medical Centre
PO Box 9101
NL–6500 HB Nijmegen (The Netherlands)
Tel. +31 24 3617203, Fax +31 24 3540251, E-Mail m.hol@kno.umcn.nl

Kompis M, Caversaccio M-D (eds): Implantable Bone Conduction Hearing Aids.
Adv Otorhinolaryngol. Basel, Karger, 2011, vol 71, pp 32–40

The Ponto Bone-Anchored Hearing System

Patrik Westerkull

Oticon Medical AB, Askim, Sweden

Abstract

Based on a foundation of a well-documented Brånemark implant experience and the most advanced sound processing technology from Oticon, Oticon Medical introduced in 2009 a new bone-anchored hearing system, the Ponto system. Although the principle of percutaneous direct bone conduction is established, new technology aiming at improving speech perception and sound comfort in noisy environments is introduced with the new Ponto system. This has been possible by using the sound-processing platform from the most advanced conventional hearing aids from Oticon. Furthermore, specific steps have been taken aiming at improving the implant as well as the skin-penetrating abutment. The Ponto sound processor coupling has been developed to withstand long-term wear and tear. With the Ponto system, a new alternative is offered to the various groups of both new and existing users of bone-anchored hearing systems. In clinical studies of the Ponto Pro sound processor, the objective testing verified the high performance of the adaptive directionality system. The subjective questionnaires on speech perception and device handling also verified that the Ponto system offers efficient hearing rehabilitation as well as other user benefits. The Ponto system also includes possibilities to fit the sound processor 2 weeks after surgery. Referred clinical studies with the Ponto system have, however, not yet been published in the literature (autumn 2010). Clinical results have this far been presented at scientific conferences.

The development of osseointegrated implants by Prof. Brånemark in the 1960s and 1970s opened up the possibility for a fixation of a direct acoustic connection to the skull bone. This sound transmission principle is referred to as direct bone conduction. Håkansson [1] demonstrated in 1984 a significant lowering of hearing thresholds, especially in the high frequencies, using direct bone conduction with skin penetration compared to traditional bone conduction across intact skin. In this experiment, Håkansson used an Oticon traditional bone conduction transducer, pressed against the skin versus when it was connected to an osseointegrated implant. Bone-anchored hearing systems based on direct bone conduction have been successfully used for more than two decades [2] offering a state of the art treatment [3] for patients with appropriate conductive or mixed hearing losses. Also patients with unilateral hearing losses are successfully helped with this technology [2].

The three main components of a bone-anchored hearing system are the screw-shaped

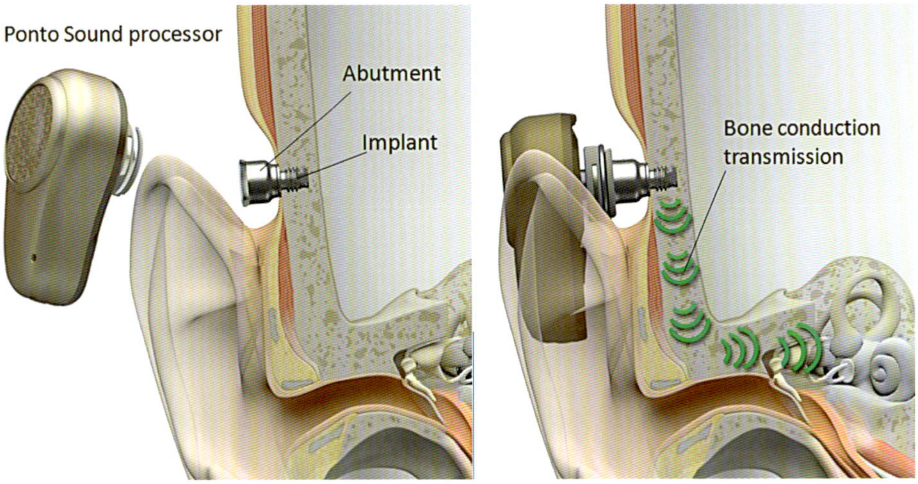

Fig. 1. When connected, the sound processor delivers bone conduction sound which is transmitted to the cochlea. (The vibrations also reach the contralateral cochlea, not shown here.)

implant which is osseointegrated in the temporal bone, the skin-penetrating abutment which is fixated to the implant with a connection screw, and the sound processor which can be connected and disconnected to the abutment. The sound processor converts sound into vibrations that are transmitted via the abutment and implant directly to the skull bones and then via direct bone conduction to the cochlea, see figure 1. The location of the abutment and the sound processor on a user can be seen in figure 2.

Despite offering significant improvements for patients with limited or no other acceptable treatment alternatives, we believe bone-anchored hearing technology has historically suffered from three primary weaknesses:

- Limited sound comfort and speech discrimination in noisy environments, primarily due to lack of advanced and appropriate signal processing, microphone systems and lack of individualized fitting programs.
- Limited durability, especially of the sound processor coupling, due to designs with small and sensitive plastic components.
- Skin irritation around the abutment, often caused by poor hygiene or a less optimal surgical approach.

An aim of the Ponto system has been to address the weaknesses listed above, as well as introducing improvements in other areas as shown below.

By gathering some of the most experienced bone-anchored hearing and implant design experts in Gothenburg, Sweden, and combining that with the sound processing and hearing aid technology and expertise of Oticon A/S of Copenhagen, Denmark, Oticon Medical has developed a new bone-anchored hearing system. The Ponto System was introduced in 2009 and includes new implants, abutments, surgical tools, advanced sound processors, fitting software and accessories. The Ponto product system is CE-marked and is cleared by the US FDA (510K No. K090996).

The Ponto implant has a Brånemark type implant surface, which is the only temporal bone implant concept for percutaneous applications with published long-term clinical data. The Ponto abutment shape and new surgical tools aim at improving skin penetration protocols and results as well as facilitating surgery.

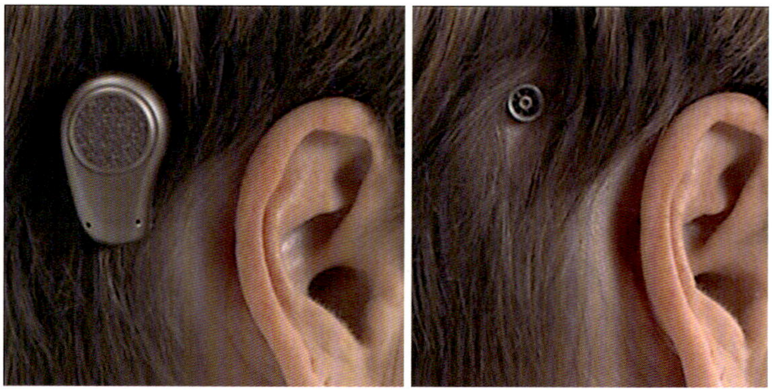

Fig. 2. Device location. To the left the Ponto sound processor is connected, and to the right the skin-penetrating abutment can be seen.

The aim of the Ponto system is to offer both existing and new users a free choice of whatever is most suitable and desired for each individual patient. Although the surgical procedure is straightforward and usually performed under local anesthesia, accepting implant surgery may represent a significant worry for the patients. Since the implant is intended to remain implanted across the lifespan, it is of significant importance to offer flexibility so that the patients can be offered an adequate device with optimal performance in different stages of their life. During their lifespan, their hearing may deteriorate, they might get a new job environment, they may need an FM accessory in school, etc. Flexibility for each patient is therefore important both regarding audiological fitting aspects as well as practical handling and aesthetics. A protocol with a procedure to use in the clinic when offering new and existing bone-anchored hearing patients the available options is very useful, and protocols like this have already been developed at some clinics [Babu, pers. commun.].

Patient Candidates

In general, patients for whom bone-anchored systems are appropriate include those with conductive hearing losses, mixed hearing losses and those with single-sided deafness.

The primary contraindication to bone-anchored hearing systems are psychiatric issues, drug and alcohol abuse and inability to maintain a hygienic abutment and surrounding skin. Indeed, poor hygiene is the chief reason for skin reactions [4].

In the USA, implantation in children below the age of 5 years is contraindicated. Small children and other patients not eligible for implantation may be helped with a Ponto sound processor attached to a softband (see below), thus allowing the device to be used as an advanced conventional bone conductor.

Audiograms and Preoperative Trial

Appropriate patients for the current Ponto and Ponto Pro sound processor models include those with bone conduction threshold (PTA based on 500, 1,000, 2,000 and 3,000 Hz) better than 45 dB HL. A new Ponto power version will be released during 2011, enabling people with greater degrees of sensorineural hearing loss component to benefit from the Ponto system.

In the case of single-sided deafness treatment, the remaining ear should have a bone conduction pure tone average better than 20 dB HL to effectively minimize head shadow effects. However, patients with somewhat more hearing loss on the 'good' ear can also often benefit from a bone-anchored device [Wazen, pers. commun.].

When considering bilateral fittings for patients with bilateral conductive or mixed hearing losses, symmetric bone conduction scores are important. The difference between the left and right bone conduction thresholds should be within 10 dB of each other with regard to pure tone average, or less than 15 dB differences at individual frequencies [5].

The Ponto system includes headbands, softbands and test rods that can be used for preoperative testing and demonstration. These accessories allow the patient to wear the device as a conventional bone conductor in their own acoustic environments for days or weeks so as to personally evaluate the benefits of bone-conducted sound. Although the preoperative trial is very important and is not to be minimized, the majority of patients report their actual bone-anchored hearing system has a better sound quality and is louder than the trial equipment [2].

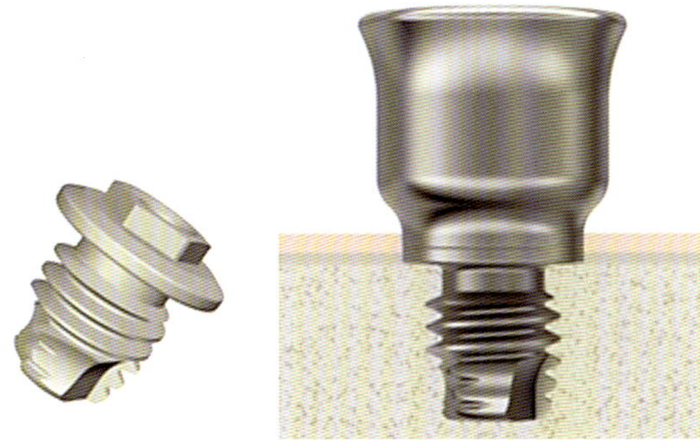

Fig. 3. Ponto implant design and abutment shape. Oticon Medical bone-anchored self-tapping titanium implant on the left, and Oticon Medical abutment design on the right.

Technology

Technology Overview

The Ponto implant system is based on a Brånemark type concept and implant surface, which has over 30 years of clinical documentation. The same surgical procedure and surgical instrumentation generally used for bone-anchored hearing aids is essentially directly applicable for the installation of the Ponto implant system, although a couple of new surgical instruments aiming at facilitating surgery is presented with the Ponto system.

The Ponto sound processors have been designed to allow individual software programming to meet the listening needs for adults and children with various needs for amplification.

Ponto's sound processors use the latest high-end sound processor chip from Oticon with automatic sound environment detectors to automatically optimize speech understanding in noise, to suppress wind noise and to incorporate microphone directionality so as to maximize the signal to noise ratio. The Ponto sound processor coupling connects on the outside of the abutment and has large contact surfaces aiming at increasing wear and tear durability of the coupling. Design, ergonomics, durability and acoustic performance have been brought together in the mechanical design of the sound processor in a multidisciplinary approach, which is important to address the need for durability, handling and feedback suppression.

Oticon Medical Implant System

The Ponto implant (see fig. 3) is self-tapping and uses a new micro-size thread design at the flange to assure maximal contact surface between the implant and the bone and discourage bone resorption. The implant has a new efficient self-tapping design that ensures an efficient engaging and optimal bone contact. The implant is available in different dimensions for different surgical preferences and the standard length is 4 mm (also available in 3 mm). The distal end of the implant is equipped with a well-documented universal Brånemark hexagon interface where the sloping part of the flange interfaces the abutment to form a conical seal. The Ponto implant is designed with a well-documented turned Brånemark type implant surface, which is the only implant surface with long-term clinical data in the temporal bone. The clinical safety and efficacy of this type of implant have been documented by, for example, Tjellström et al. [6]. Although various surface treatments and surfaces of different roughness are used among dental implants, there is no evidence in the literature showing that any particular type of the established dental implants has superior long-term success [7]. The only statistically significant finding in the literature was that more implants with rough surfaces were affected by inflammatory response (peri-implantitis) at the bone surface compared to the turned Brånemark type of surfaces [7]. A rough surface offers additional surface for biofilm formation and bacterial adhesion, and considering the proximity to the skin penetration we believe it is not beneficiary to have rough surfaces at the upper part of the implant where it may interact with the skin penetration. Although osseointegration of the implant is rarely a challenge with any bone-anchored hearing system, implant development is an ongoing activity.

Skin penetration is, however, a critical concern for bone-anchored hearing systems. Therefore, it is important to try to optimize the skin-penetrating components and the surgical skin preparation to ensure a long-term reaction free skin penetration. The Oticon Medical implant and abutment are designed to ensure that the skin can be fully supported and fixated by the underlying bone and periosteum – all the way to the abutment without having unsupported skin in a circular groove or on top of the implant flange. Thus, as skin movement is minimized, this design aims at minimizing postoperative local infection and irritation. Skin movement in relation to the abutment can be a cause for skin irritation [4]. The conical design located at the interface between the implant and abutment forms a tight seal between the components, to avoid bacterial leakage between the components. In figure 3, the Ponto implant components are shown. The Oticon Medical implant and abutment include no magnetic or ferromagnetic materials. Titanium implants without ferromagnetic materials have been documented to be compatible with magnetic resonance imaging [8].

Oticon Medical abutments are available in different lengths, although the 6 mm and 9 mm lengths are the most commonly used. An angled abutment (10°) is also available as an option for correction on patients where the implant could not be placed in an optimal orientation due to, for example, anatomic variations. Correct orientation of the device may help to avoid feedback in cases where the device touches the skin or the pinna. Correct orientation is also important for optimal directional microphone orientation as well as aesthetics.

Surgical Procedure and Implant Healing

For osseointegrating implants in general, it is important that the implant should not be mobile in relation to the bone during the osseointegration process. High loads on the implant during the healing may lead to movements, which may jeopardize osseointegration. No minimal time between implant insertion of a Brånemark type implant and fitting of the sound processor has been documented. In adults with normal bone, the sound processor can be safely fitted 6 weeks after implantation [9], but there are also clinics that are successfully fitting the devices after 4 weeks [Somers, pers. commun.]. Initial implant stability as well as patient-related factors should be considered when deciding when the sound processor may be fitted. In small children with soft bone, a two-stage surgical procedure and a significantly longer time for osseointegration should be applied prior to fitting [4].

At normal use, the highest forces that the implant is exposed to are when the sound processor is connected and disconnected from the abutment. In cases where it is desirable to significantly

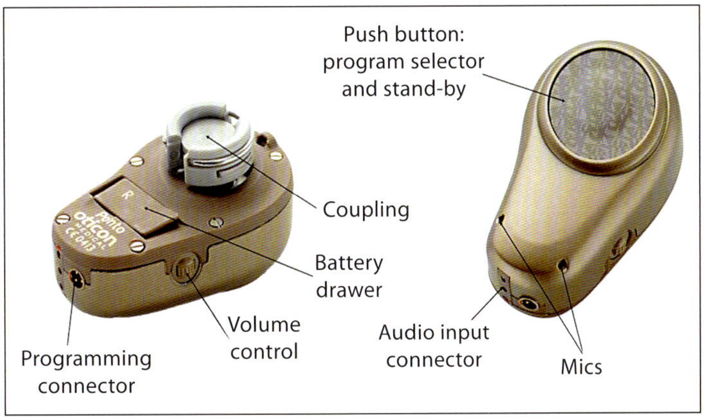

Fig. 4. Ponto sound processors with the coupling, connectors and controls marked. The devices are available in left and right versions and multiple colors.

reduce this connection and disconnection force, the Ponto Xpress accessory may be used. The Xpress is an interconnection unit with control handles that can be connected to the sound processor coupling so that the device can be connected and disconnected without any significant forces on the implant. This may, for example, be useful in situations where the surgeon considers there might be a risk for implant mobility with regular coupling forces during the healing period, but in which the patient still needs the device, see also clinical results below.

The Ponto surgical procedure is in line with established surgical procedures for bone-anchored hearing systems. Thick skin up around the upper portion of the abutment should always be avoided for bone-anchored hearing aids since this may be a reason for skin irritation [4] and this may also interfere with the Ponto coupling. In the case of thick skin up around the abutment, a longer abutment or possibly a skin revision surgery should be applied.

The same surgical instrumentation used for any bone-anchored hearing aid surgery can be used also with the Ponto system. However, some new instrument developments come with the Ponto system. One example of new surgical tool developed by Oticon Medical together with the Swiss company Nouvag is a new dermatome (Ref. No. 1994 NOU) with adjustable flap thickness (0.6–1.0 mm) and blade side pads to ensure straight precision cut edges.

Ponto Processors and Accessories

There are currently (autumn 2010) two processor models, Ponto and Ponto Pro. The shape and mechanics are identical for the two models, and both are based on the same electronic hardware. However, the Ponto Pro includes software for more sophisticated automatic signal processing than the Ponto model. Both models include, for example, wind noise detector with automatic suppression, multiband adaptive directionality, output compression, 10-channel frequency shaping and up to 4 programs. Features currently unique to Ponto Pro include: tri-state noise reduction, learning volume control, data logging and an automatic 3-mode control of the directionality. The Ponto model can manually be switched between omnidirectional and directional modes. Both models can be individually fitted and programmed using the Genie Medical fitting software, and both models are available in left and right designs, shaped to offer practical handling, good ergonomics and aesthetics. The Ponto device can be seen in figure 4.

The adaptive directionality system of the Ponto and Ponto Pro detects the angle of the dominant noise source and automatically changes the polar pattern to provide maximum attenuation for that noise. The benefit of the adaptive directionality may be especially important for bone-anchored hearing aids, since the microphone position here is usually less optimal than for a conventional air conduction hearing aid.

Ponto Pro is also currently the only bone-anchored sound processor on the market that includes tri-state noise reduction with speech detector and modulation detector. The device can therefore detect if it is a situation with speech in quiet, speech in noise or a situation with noise only. The Ponto Pro can then adapt the noise reduction in each channel to maximize speech understanding in each listening situation.

In addition to the Ponto and Ponto Pro models, a Ponto Power device will be available during the first half of 2011. This new device will have all the features of the Ponto Pro, as well as additional advanced fitting and processing options, especially suitable for power device users.

The Genie Medical fitting software is designed in accordance with the concept of the established Oticon Genie fitting software, and we believe therefore it is intuitive and easy to operate for the audiologists. Prescriptions are usually derived from the entered left and right bone conduction thresholds.

There are a several accessories available for the Ponto Processors, such as an FM receiver, an audio adapter, etc. For very young children and for patients ineligible for implantation, the sound processor can be connected to the Softband. The Softband is an elastic band with a connection for the sound processor, so that it can be used as a conventional bone conductor. The Softband has a built in safety release mechanism and can also easily be used for bilateral fittings.

Ponto and Ponto Pro Coupling

The sound processor coupling is a key to durability and the ability to withstand extensive wear and tear. The coupling includes separate contact material and spring materials. The metal spring ensures long-term spring function and the polymer contact material is designed with generous contact surfaces and ensures long-term durability, high performance sound transmission and user-friendly handling. Big contact surfaces between the abutment and the coupling at the connection of the device are a critical design factor determining durability of the coupling, since small contact surfaces are worn out more easily.

Clinical Results

In two studies presented by Olsen et al. [10, 11], the objective and subjective outcome of the Ponto Pro sound processor was studied. The study included 12 patients with a median observation period of 34 days. In the objective measurements, the Ponto Pro was tested in terms of speech recognition thresholds in noise. In this test with speech (DANTALE II) [12] from 0° and noise from ±90°, the efficiency of the directional microphone system of the Ponto Pro was demonstrated. The Ponto Pro is currently the only bone-anchored processor on the market with automatic 3-mode adaptive directionality. Since the directionality of the Ponto Pro is adaptive when the device is set in directional mode, it can suppress noise coming from the side more efficiently than a device with fixed directionality, where the minimum sensitivity of the directional microphone is fixed and usually from behind (see fig. 5). Speech perception in various listening situations was also subjectively evaluated with the NSH (Nordic cooperation on disability) questionnaire. On this 1–10 scale where 10 is the best rating, Ponto Pro scored between 6 and 8.5 in the various listening situations, which can be regarded as a very good rating. Another reason for this high patient rating on speech perception may be that the Ponto Pro does not only have an omnidirectional and a directional mode, but it has also a split directional mode where the device is in omni mode for low frequencies and in directional mode for higher frequencies. The split directional mode is frequently used in many daily situations where neither full directional nor

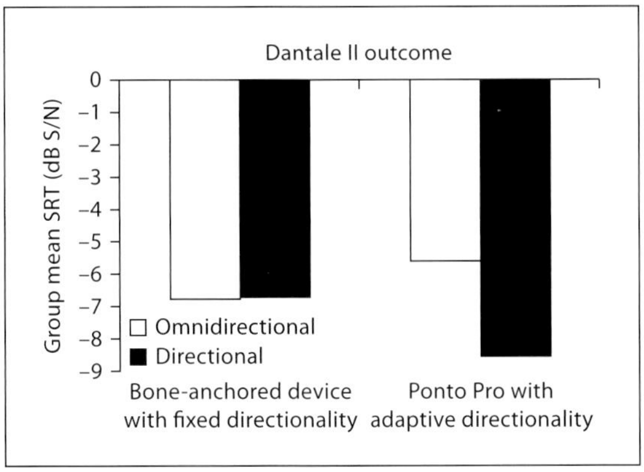

Fig. 5. Speech recognition thresholds (SRT) in noise. Speech presented from 0° and noise from ±90° (n = 10). From study by Olsen et al. [11]. DANTALE II from Wagener et al. [12].

omni mode is optimal. The Ponto Pro is currently the only bone-anchored sound processor on the market that offers a 3-mode adaptive directionality. A third reason for the high rating may be that the Ponto Pro has a tri-state noise reduction system, see above. In this study, also the ease of handling was investigated using the NSH questionnaires. On this 1–10 scale where 10 is the best rating, Ponto Pro scored around 8–9 on all aspects, which can be regarded as a very good result. The complete presentation from this study can be viewed at the website of the Danish technical audiological society (www.dtas.info).

In two separate studies presented by Reid et al. [13] and Granström [14], results from clinical studies of the Ponto implant system and the Xpress accessory have been presented. The studies included 9 and 8 patients, respectively, who underwent regular Ponto surgery. A Ponto sound processor with an Xpress accessory was fitted 2 weeks after surgery, so that the patient could start to benefit from the device. After an additional 6 weeks, the Xpress accessory was removed, and the sound processor was then connected to the abutment in the regular way. No implant losses occurred during the 12-month follow-up.

Several ongoing clinical studies will add to the scientific documentation of the safety and efficacy of the Ponto implant system and the Ponto sound processors.

Discussion and Conclusion

Bone-anchored hearing systems have been available for more than two decades, and have been built upon a solid foundation of scientific and clinical outcomes demonstrating undeniable benefits for many patient groups. Beyond the primary goal of improved hearing, bone-anchored systems have contributed to improvements in behavior, concentration, learning and development in children [15].

The Ponto system provides a next step in advanced bone-anchored hearing systems, thereby positioning Oticon Medical's Bone Anchored Hearing System as an efficient new choice for appropriate candidates.

In clinical testing, the Ponto Pro sound processor scored very well in both objective speech in noise testing as well as in subjective questions on speech perceptions and practical handling of the device. The conclusion from this is that the Ponto Pro offers improvements on several aspects and that the Ponto Pro offers efficient hearing rehabilitation as well as a user-friendly and safe treatment.

The Ponto system is based on a well-documented implant concept with new developments aiming at further improving also the surgical side. The Ponto system also includes possibilities to fit the sound processor 2 weeks after surgery.

Further clinical studies will be performed and are also underway from clinics around the world.

Even if the Ponto system is a significant step forward in bone-anchored hearing, there is still plenty of room for further improvements in the field of bone-anchored hearing systems.

References

1 Håkansson B, Tjellström A, Rosenhall U: Hearing thresholds with direct bone conduction versus conventional bone conduction. Scand Audiol 1984;12: 3–13.

2 Snik AF, Mylanus EAM, Proops DW, Wolfaardt JF, Dent M, Hodgetts WE, Somers T, Niparko JK, Wazen JJ, Sterkers O, Cremers CWRJ, Tjellstrom A: Consensus Statement on the BAHA System: where do we stand at present? Ann Otol Rhinol Laryngol 2005; 114(suppl):1–12.

3 Snik AFM, Bosman AJ, Mylanus EAM, Cremers CWRJ: Candidacy for the bone-anchored hearing aid. Audiol Neurootol 2004;9:190–196.

4 Tjellstrom A, Hakansson B, Granstrom G: Bone-anchored hearing aids; in Maniglia AJ, Proops DW (eds): Implantable Electronic Otologic Devices – State of the Art. Otolaryngol Clin North Am. Philadelphia, WB Saunders, 2001, vol 34.

5 Bosman AJ, Snik AF, van der Pouw CT, Mylanus EA, Cremers CWRJ: Audiometric evaluation of bilaterally fitted bone-anchored hearing aids. Audiology 2001;40:158–176.

6 Tjellstrom A, Hakansson B, Granstrom G, Odersjö M: Survival rate of self-tapping implants for bone-anchored hearing aids. J Laryngol Otol 2007;121: 101–104.

7 Palmquist A, Omar M, Esposito M, Lausmaa J, Thomsen P: Titanium oral implants: surface characteristics, interface biology and clinical outcome. J R Soc Interface 2010;7(suppl 5): S515–S527.

8 Devge C, Tjellström A, Nellström H: Magnetic resonance imaging in patients with dental implants: a clinical report. Int J Oral Max Impl 1997;12:354–359.

9 Wazen J, Gupta R, Ghossaini S, Spitzer JB, Farrugia M, Tjellstrom A: Osseointegration timing for Baha system loading. Laryngoscope DOI: 10.1097/01.mlg.0000231281.76358.cc.

10 Olsen SØ, Glad H, Nielsen LH: Comparison of two newly introduced bone anchored hearing instruments in ten first-time users; in 11th Int Conf Cochlear Implants, Stockholm, June 2010.

11 Olsen SØ, Glad H, Nielsen LH: Comparison of two newly introduced bone anchored hearing instruments in first-time users, updated September 2010; in DTAS (Danish Technical Audiological Society) Annu Meet, Vejle, September 2010.

12 Wagener K, Josvassen JL, Ardenkjaer R: Design, optimization and evaluation of a Danish sentence test in noise. Int J Audiol 2003;42:10–17.

13 Reid AP, Proops D, Burell S, Egan E: Clinical study of an interconnection unit for earlier fitting access of a bone anchored hearing aid; in 2nd Int Symp Bone Conduction, Göteborg, June 2009.

14 Granström G: Xpress coupling for bone conduction hearing devices (poster); 11th Int Conference Cochlear Implants, Stockholm, June 2010.

15 McDermott AL, Williams J, Kuo MJ, Reid A, Proops D: Quality of life in children fitted with a bone anchored hearing aid. Otol Neurotol 2009;30:344–349.

Patrik Westerkull, MSc Eng Ph
Oticon Medical AB
Ekonomiv 2
SE–43633 Askim (Sweden)
Tel. +46 317486100, Fax +46 31687756, E-Mail paw@oticonmedical.se

Kompis M, Caversaccio M-D (eds): Implantable Bone Conduction Hearing Aids.
Adv Otorhinolaryngol. Basel, Karger, 2011, vol 71, pp 41–46

Partially Implantable Bone Conduction Hearing Aids without a Percutaneous Abutment (Otomag): Technique and Preliminary Clinical Results

Ralf Siegert

Department of Oto-Rhino-Laryngology, Head and Neck Surgery, Recklinghausen, Germany

Abstract

Introduction: Patients with air-bone gaps who cannot be corrected successfully by tympanoplasty or with mixed hearing loss may be treated with bone conduction hearing aids. Their disadvantages are the obvious external fixation components or the biological and psychosocial problems of open implants. We have developed new partially implantable bone conduction hearing aid without a percutaneous abutment and have been using them clinically for 4 years. The principle of these bone conduction hearing aids is a magnetic coupling and acoustic transmission between implanted and external magnets. The goal of this study was to evaluate clinical and audiological results. **Methods:** Magnets are implanted into shallow bone beds in a one step procedure. The skin above the magnets is also reduced to a thickness of 4–5 mm, which reduces the attenuation to less than 10 dB compared to direct bone stimulation. Over 100 patients have been implanted in the last 5 years. **Results:** Except for temporary pressure marks in 4%, which healed after careful shimming of the external base plate, there were no other complications. **Discussion:** The holding strength of the external components is equivalent to partially implantable hearing aids and cochlea implants and the hearing improvement is similar to other bone conduction hearing aids. We have found the comfort and safety of this system is significantly improved compared to conventional or percutaneous bone conduction hearing aids.

Patients with air-bone gaps that cannot be corrected successfully by tympanoplasty or with mixed hearing loss may be treated with bone conduction hearing aids (BCHA). Three options have been used clinically to transmit the sound into the bone; two of them are still available.

1 Conventional BCHA: In conventional BCHA, a vibrator is pressed onto the skin above the mastoid with a headband or an elastic arch [1]. The sound energy is transmitted through the skin into the bone and from there on – almost without any further attenuation – into the cochlea. Their disadvantages are the pressure applied to the skin and the conspicuousness of the external components.

2 Bone-anchored hearing aids (Baha): Baha have been used clinically since 30 years [2–4]. The Baha allows a direct sound conduction via an abutment, which is fixed to the temporal bone and perforates the skin. The Baha disadvantages

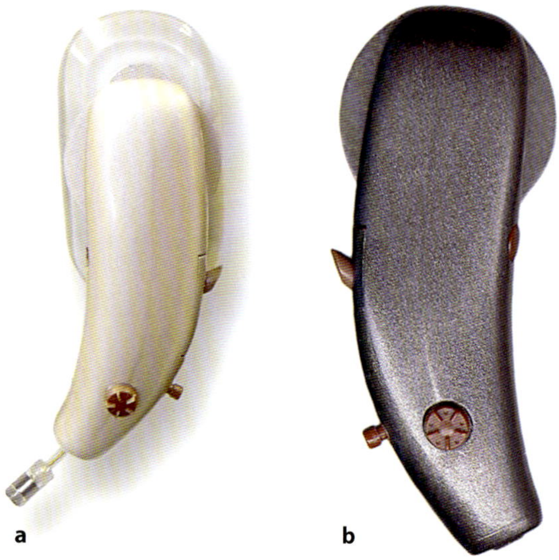

Fig. 1. External components of this partially implantable bone conduction aid with (**a**) and without (**b**) baseplate in different colors.

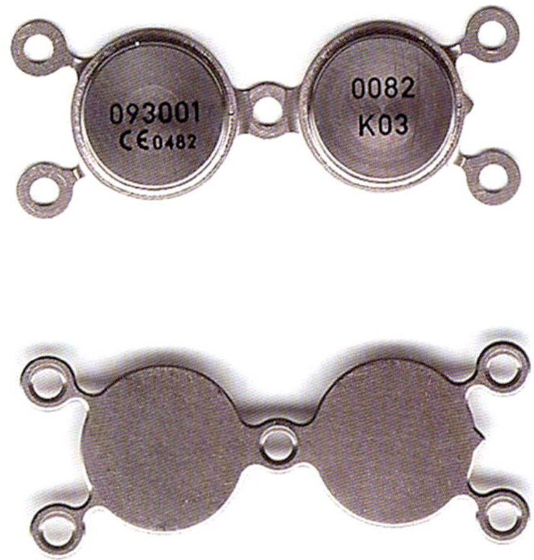

Fig. 2. Implantable twin magnet (Otomag).

are the biological and psychosocial problems of the percutaneous abutment with the risk of inflammation and injuries and the necessity of more than one operation [5, 6].

3 Partially implantable bone conduction hearing aids with electromagnetic energy transmission (Audiant): To avoid the disadvantages of open implants, an electromagnetic induction technique with an implanted vibrator has been used for some time. Although vibrations could really be transmitted into the skull, its amplification was too low, and its energy consumption was much too high for routine clinical use [7, 8]. This system is not available any more.

Due to the mentioned disadvantages, there was a need to optimize bone conduction hearing systems. The goals of this project were to develop (1) a new partially implantable bone conduction hearing system without a percutaneous abutment, (2) the surgical technique for its implantation, (3) its postoperative adjustment, and (4) the clinical introduction of this system.

Material and Methods

The Partially Implantable Bone Conduction Hearing Device

The principle of these new bone conduction hearing devices is the magnetic coupling between implanted and external magnets [9]. To reduce the magnetic perturbations of the vibrator and provide rotational stability, a magnetic circle with 4 high-strength magnets is constructed (fig. 1). The implantable twin magnets are made out of samarium-cobalt encapsulated in a titanium case with little arms like bone plates to fix the implant with screws (fig. 2).

The external twin magnets have a similar geometry as the implanted ones. They are embedded into an acrylic base plate, which is firmly connected with the vibrator.

The vibrator is controlled by a fully digital, 4-channel processor with 16 frequency bands, adaptive noise reduction and 5 adjustable notch filters. The omnidirectional microphone, battery (type 675, operating time ca. 630 h), chip and vibrator (280–5,400 Hz) are built in an acrylic housing in the standard version (Otomag). For special requirements, the microphone can be placed outside of this housing or exchanged to a directional microphone.

In addition to an air-bone gap, patients with a mixed hearing loss (with an up to 40-dB sensorineural component) as well as single-sided deafness patients may be treated with this device.

Surgical Technique
The twin magnets can be implanted under general or local anesthesia. A curved incision approximately 7 cm behind and above (superior and posterior) the external ear canal is performed all the way down to the bone. After exposure of an area of about 30 × 15 mm, the implant is positioned 6 cm away from the external ear canal and the bone marked with a pen (fig. 3a). Then, shallow bone beds are drilled out with a depth of at least 2.6 mm for the magnets (fig. 3b). The implant is then placed into these bone beds (fig. 3c) and fixed with mini-screws (e.g. diameter 1.5 mm; Martin; fig. 3d).

Finally, the skin above the magnets is thinned out to a thickness of 4–5 mm, which reduces the relatively high attenuation in conventional BCHA to less than 10 dB compared to direct bone stimulation. To measure the skin thickness, a fork-like instrument (Grosse; fig. 3e) has been constructed. The incision is closed with fast resorbable sutures which do not need to be removed in the hair-bearing area. A small pressure bandage is applied for one day.

Patients
After approval by the local ethics committee (Ruhr-Universität Bochum, AZ: 2589 from 04.10.2005) the first implantation was performed on the 31.01.2006. Since then, implantations in >100 patients have been performed. Most of them had a conductive hearing loss due to congenital auricular atresia. These were patients with severe middle ear malformations that could not be corrected by tympanoplasty [10–12].

Before implantation, all patients tried bone conduction amplification via a bite block analogue to the procedure before Baha implantation.

All patients (and in minors also their parents) were informed extensively about this study as well as the alternatives of conventional BCHA and Baha. In addition, they were informed that MRI is not allowed as long as the magnets are in place. Alternatively, they could have CT or a temporary explantation of the magnets possibly under local anesthesia.

Fitting of the Hearing Aids
After one month, the external base plate with the counter magnets is adjusted and the hearing aids fitted individually with the Optifit software similar to other digital hearing aids.

Results

Clinical Follow-Up

No complications related to the implantation were observed. All wounds healed uneventfully. In some cases, slight pressure marks occurred, which healed after careful shimming and slight force reduction of the base plates. The hearing aids are very inconspicuous (fig. 4).

The clinical and audiological follow-up is ongoing. Detailed, but preliminary results of 12 patients (8 unilateral, 4 bilateral) showed an average skin thickness over the implants of 3.8 ± 0.5 mm and a holding strength of the base plates chosen by the patients of 0.8 ± 0.4 N.

The average hearing gain in free field pure tone audiogram was 31.2 ± 8.1 dB and the suprathreshold speech perception at 65 dB in free field increased from 12.9 without to 72.1% with the hearing device.

Discussion

BCHA may be indicated in the following situations: (1) Severe air bone gap or combined hearing loss. BCHA are especially necessary in situations where tympanoplasty is not successful in the long-term, like in severe middle ear malformation with unfavorable anatomic conditions [10] or chronic sclerosing otitis. (2) Single-sided deafness (SSD). In SSD, BCHA are an alternative to CROSS systems [13, 14]. (3) Sensorineural hearing loss which cannot be treated with conventional hearing aids. Problems with the 'classic' air conduction hearing aid can occur in chronic external otitis, wet external ear canals from inside due to otorrhea, from outside due to perspiration, rain (e.g. in gardeners) or other difficult environmental conditions (e.g. cooks). (4) Psychological aspects. BCHA worn behind the ear in the hair-bearing area are less visible.

As mentioned before, there are two different bone conduction systems on the market:
- Conventional BCHA with a vibrator, which is pressed onto the retroauricular skin by a headband or a similar device.
- BCHA which transmit the sound through a percutaneous abutment into the bone.

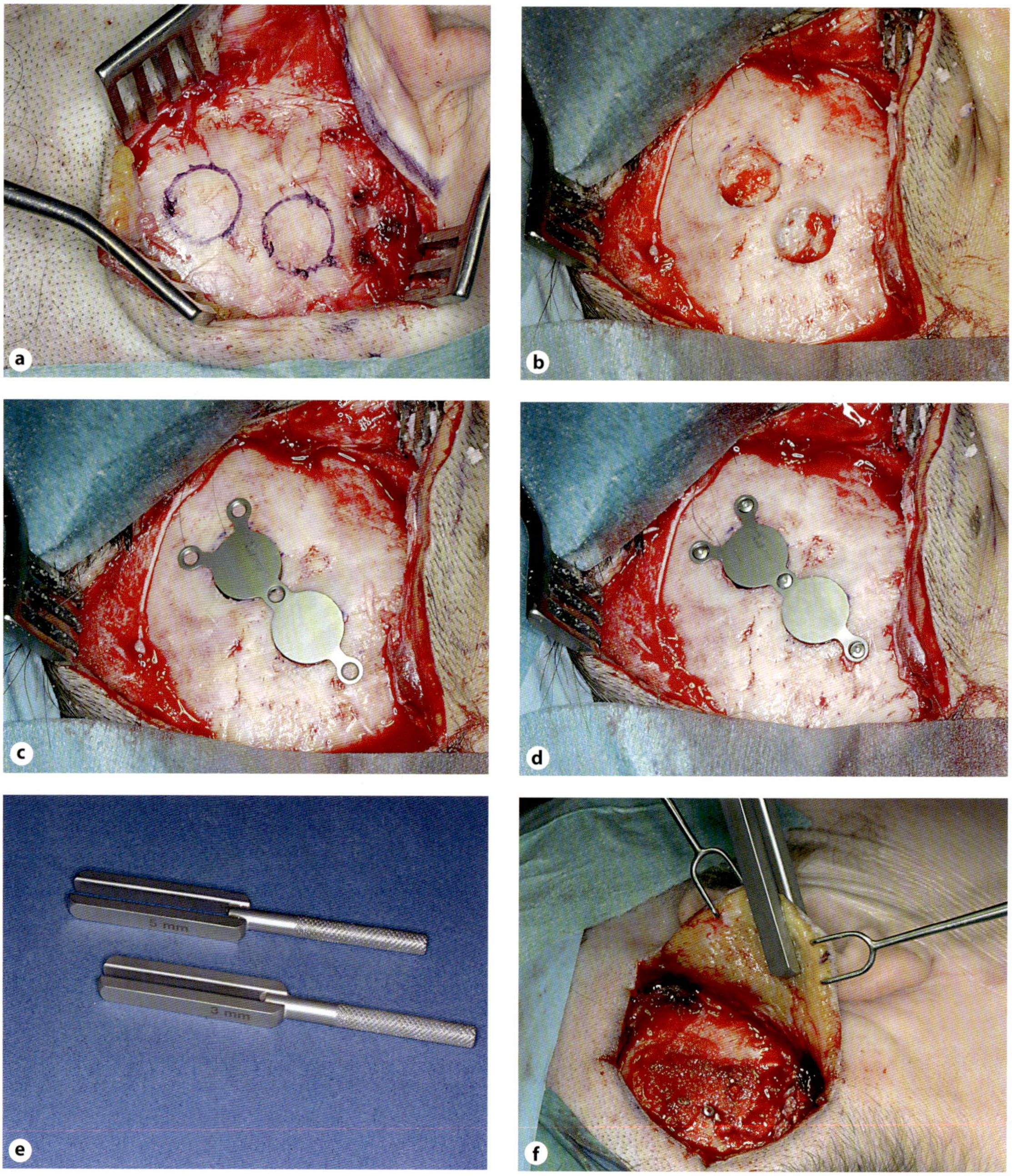

Fig. 3. Implantation of the magnets. **a** Markings for the position of the implantable magnet on the mastoid. **b** Bone beds with a depth of at least 2.6 mm for the magnets. **c** Twin magnet in place. **d** Twin magnet fixed with 4 bone microscrews. **e** Device to measure the skin thickness; 5 mm (top) and 3 mm (bottom). **f** Intraoperative measurement of the skin thickness.

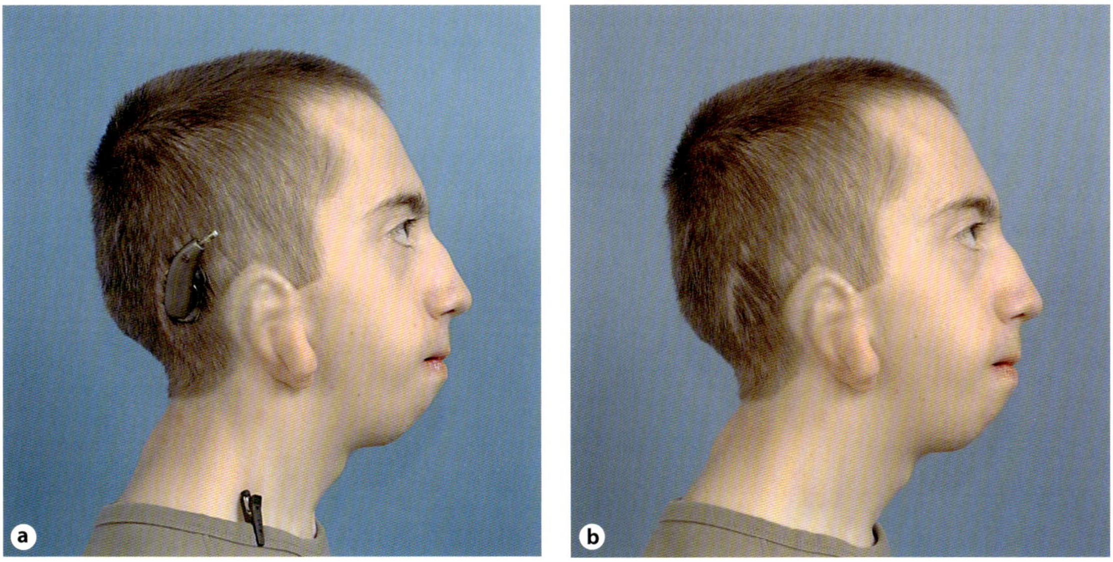

Fig. 4. Patient (after first step of ongoing auricular reconstruction) with his magnetically fixed BCHA with (**a**) without (**b**) external device in place.

Both systems have the disadvantages mentioned above. Here, we present a new principle of a BCHA. It is partially implantable, fixed to the head by magnets and transmits the sound through the intact, but slightly thinned out skin into the bone.

After a variety of lab tests and approval of the local ethics committee, the first implantation was performed on the 31.01.2006. Since then, >100 implantations have been done without any intraoperative or postoperative complications.

The wearing comfort of this new system is very good. The patient does not need a headband or an abutment. Instead, the implants, scars and external components are hidden under the skin by hair. No hair or hair follicles have to be removed. If the patients take their hearing processors off, they can do all physical activities as before. There is no increased risk for injury, whether for themselves or their sports partner.

For daily life activities, the holding strength is sufficient. It is basically the same as for the external components of cochlear implants that have been in use for decades. In addition, the base plates can be changed by the patient himself easily so that he or she can wear stronger ones for sport activities and weaker ones for quiescent situations.

The sound processors have to be fitted in the more or less typical way. Its digital processor and the software allow for multiple individualized adjustments. The sound attenuation caused by the intact, thinned skin as measured in the previous lab test is less than 10 dB compared to direct bone coupling as in Baha. This can be compensated for easily in the majority of patients with only minor sensorineural hearing loss in addition to an air-bone gap.

According to our experiences up to now, this system can be characterized by the following aspects: (1) only one, relatively easy and fast operation, (2) no wound healing or pressure complications, (3) no biological or psychological problems related to percutaneous abutments, (4) no external pressure by a headband, (5) good wearing comfort, (6) a hearing gain, which is comparable to the other BCHA.

Therefore, we think that patients who need BCHA should be informed about this option as a third choice beside conventional BCHA and Baha.

Disclosure Statement

The presented principle and the new BCHA were developed by the author in cooperation with Otomag. The project was sponsored by Arbeitsgemeinschaft industrieller Forschungsvereinigungen 'Otto von Guericke' e.V.

References

1 Mylanus EAM, van der Pouw CTM, Snik AFM, Cremers WRJ: Intraindividual comparison of the bone-anchored hearing aid and air-conduction hearing aids. Arch Otolaryngol 1998;124: 271–276.

2 Tjellström A, Hakansson B: The bone-anchored hearing aid. Otolaryngol Clin North Am 1995;28:53–72.

3 Papsin BC, Sirimanna TKS, Albert DM, Bailey CM: Surgical experience with bone-anchored hearing aids in children. Laryngoscope 1997;107:801–806.

4 Snik AF, Mylanus EA, Proops DW, Wolfaardt JF, Hodgetts WE, Somers T, Niparko JK, Wazen JJ, Sterkers O, Cremers CW, Tjellström A: Consensus statements on the BAHA system: where do we stand at present? Ann Otol Rhino Laryngol 2005;195(suppl):2–12.

5 Zeitoun H, De R, Thomson SD, Proops DW: Difficulties with bone anchored hearing aids in children. J Laryngol Otol 2002;116:87–91.

6 Shirazi MA, Marzo SJ, Leonetti JP: Perioperative complications with the bone-anchored hearing aid. Otolaryngol Head Neck Surg 2006;134:236–239.

7 Hough JV, Hough DA, McGee M: Long-term results for the Xomed Audiant Bone Conductor. Otolaryngol Clin North Am 1995;28:43–52.

8 Håkansson B, Tjellström A, Carlsson P: Percutaneous vs. transcutaneous transducers for hearing by direct bone conduction. Otolaryngol Head Neck Surg 1990;102:339–344.

9 Siegert R: Knochenleitungshörgerät mit Doppelmagnetankopplung. DBGM 20 2005 009 361.0, 2005.

10 Siegert R, Weerda H, Mayer T, Brückmann H: Hochauflösende Computertomographie fehlgebildeter Mittelohren. Laryngorhinootologie 1996;75:187–194.

11 Siegert R: The combined reconstruction of congenital auricular atresia and severe microtia. Laryngoscope 2003;113: 2021–2029.

12 Siegert R: Neue Wege bei der chirurgischen Behandlung der kongenitalen Gehörgangsatresie. HNO 2004;52: 275–288.

13 Wazen JJ, Spitzer JB, Ghossaini SN, Fayad JN, Niparko JK, Cox K, Brackmann DE, Soli SD: Transcranial contralateral cochlear stimulation in unilateral deafness. Otolaryngol Head Neck Surg 2003;129:248–254.

14 Hol MK, Bosman AJ, Snik AF, Mylanus EA, Cremers CW: Bone-anchored hearing aids in unilateral inner ear deafness: an evaluation of audiometric and patient outcome measurements. Otol Neurotol 2005;26:999–1006.

Prof. Dr. Dr. Ralf Siegert
Department of Oto-Rhino-Laryngology, Head and Neck Surgery, Prosper Hospital
Muehlenstrasse 27
DE–45659 Recklinghausen (Germany)
Tel. +49 2361 54 2550, Fax +49 2361 54 2590, E-Mail profsiegert@web.de

Kompis M, Caversaccio M-D (eds): Implantable Bone Conduction Hearing Aids.
Adv Otorhinolaryngol. Basel, Karger, 2011, vol 71, pp 47–55

Surgery for the Bone-Anchored Hearing Aid

Andreas Arnold[a] · Marco-Domenico Caversaccio[a] · Albert Mudry[b]

[a]Department of ENT, Head and Neck Surgery, Inselspital, University of Bern, Bern, [b]ENT and HNS, Lausanne, Switzerland

Abstract

Introduction: This review covers the surgery for the bone-anchored hearing aid (Baha®). **Preoperative Workup:** A review of the indications and preoperative diagnostics shows that best results are generally obtained in patients with conductive or mixed hearing loss rehabilitation when surgery is not applicable or has failed and in patients that suffer from single-sided deafness. An audiogram must confirm that the bone conduction hearing is within the inclusion criteria. A computed tomography scan is performed in cases of malformation to assure sufficient bone thickness at the site of screw implantation. **Procedure:** The steps of the Baha implantation are described step by step including the setting and anesthesia, skin work with regard to different techniques, correct resection of subcutaneous tissue, preparation of the implant site, drilling and placement of the fixture and wound closure. **Postoperative Care:** After wound healing (6–8 weeks), the bone conduction aid is fitted on the abutment. Regular cleaning of the fixture is important to avoid irritations and infections. **Conclusion:** If performed carefully, the surgery for the Baha has a favorable outcome, regardless of the technique used.

The surgical placement of the bone-anchored hearing aid (Baha®) is a procedure where detailed care has to be taken in all steps of the implantation [1]. Especially the work on the skin surrounding the titanium implant deserves attention to avoid a delay in healing and later skin overgrowth or even chronic inflammation. Furthermore, precise drilling and placement of the titanium fixture in the temporal bone is paramount to accomplish firm osseointegration.

Since 1992, the centers of Berne and Lausanne have gained experience in surgery for the Baha. Up to now, 501 Baha implantations, of which 100 in children, have been performed.

This chapter briefly reviews the indications, preoperative diagnostics, setting and anesthesia. Subsequently, all steps of the implantation procedure are described, including the different skin approaches (skin flap techniques, linear incision technique), the necessary soft tissue work and the placement of the screw, wound closure and postoperative care.

Indications

The two major indications for an implantable bone conduction hearing aid are conductive or mixed hearing loss rehabilitation when surgery is not applicable or has failed and single-sided deafness (SSD).

The first group comprises ears with chronic secretion not allowing adaptation of conventional

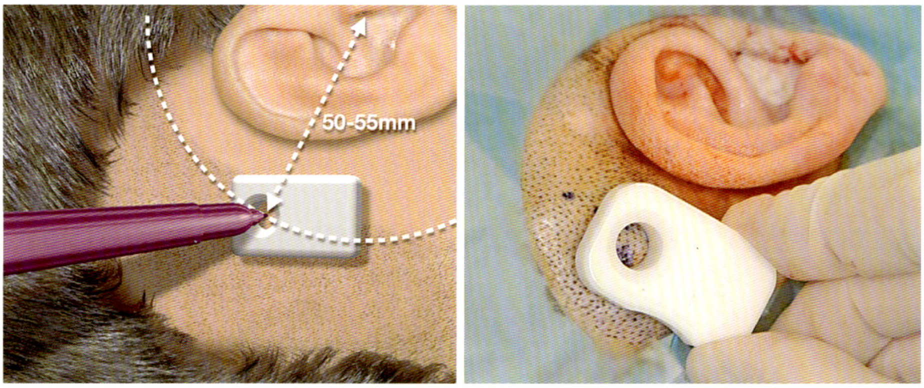

Fig. 1. The site of incision is marked with a pen with the help of the template from the implantation set.

hearing aids (e.g. chronic otits externa, eczema, chronic middle ear infections), congenital malformations of external and/or middle ear (external/middle ear atresia, craniofacial malformations) and patients unsatisfied with hearing aids or other bone conduction devices.

The second group includes patients that have a complete or nearly complete SSD due to, for example, vestibular schwannoma surgery, middle ear surgery (stapedectomy), sudden hearing loss or congenital deafness. These patients are fitted with a bone conduction hearing aid on the deaf side, and the signal is routed via the patient's skull to the contralateral normal hearing ear. This fitting is therefore referred to as contralateral routing of signal (CROS). Wazen et al. [2] showed better speech intelligibility in SSD patients with a CROS fitting due to a reduction in the acoustical head shadow.

Preoperative Diagnostics

The diagnostic workup before surgery must assure that the patient's bone conduction hearing meets the inclusion criteria for a bone conduction hearing aid and, at least in case of malformations, that the patient's temporal bone thickness is sufficient to allow a safe implantation of the device. Therefore, an audiological assessment includes a pure tone audiogram with bone conduction, as well as a speech audiogram.

A high-resolution computed tomography scan of the temporal bones is performed in cases where a sufficient bone thickness is questionable at the site of the screw implantation.

For the audiological criteria for Baha implantation that assure a high patient benefit refer to the chapters in the section 'Audiological Aspects'.

Setting and Anesthesia

Since the mid-1990s, the implantation of the Baha is usually performed as a one-stage procedure. The surgery is performed in an operating room with regular sterility precautions. The procedure is performed under local anesthesia in adults and general anesthesia in children.

A small amount of hair behind and above the ear of the side to be implanted has to be shaved. After injection of the local anesthesia (4–8 ml of Xylocaine 2% with adrenaline), the site of incision is marked with a pen with the help of the template from the implantation set (fig. 1). The site to place the screw is retroauricularly upward of the lateral sinus curve. The implantation site on

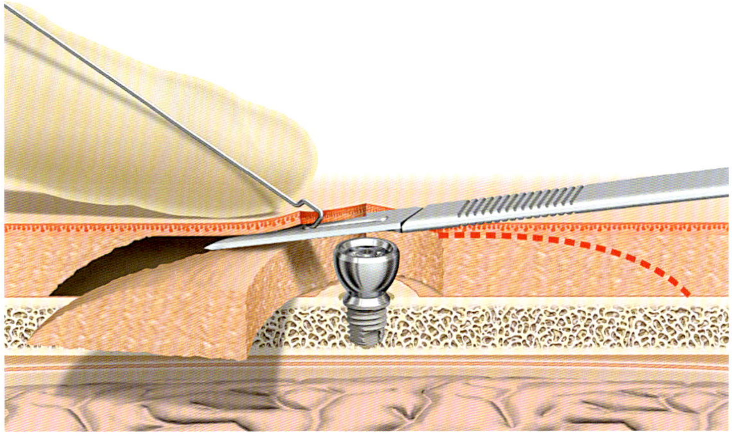

Fig. 2. A large area of SCT is resected at the skin borders in an outward angle to minimize tissue bulk above and around the screw implantation site.

the periosteum can be marked using a needle with blue dye stitched through the skin before incision to avoid wrong positioning of the implant after elevation of the flap.

Skin and Soft Tissue Work

The skin incision depends on the approach chosen. Independent of the incision technique, it is paramount that a large area of subcutaneous tissue (SCT) is resected at the skin borders in an outward angle to minimize tissue bulk above and around the screw implantation site (fig. 2). Skin undermining and SCT resection are recommended to be at least 25 mm in every direction [3].

In all cases where the cutaneous flap is not lifted with an electric dermatome, the underside of the skin has to be totally cleared from hair follicles using a fresh blade. The SCT resection and skin follicle removal is the most significant part of the soft tissue work as it prevents the overgrowth of hair and skin during wound healing as well as later inflammatory complications.

After resection of the SCT, the periosteum of the mastoid plane is exposed.

The periosteum is incised crosswise and pulled aside using a small rasparatory. The periosteum is preserved except at the screw implantation site.

Alternatives in Skin and Soft Tissue Procedures

Rectangle Flap (Dermatome)
A square cutaneous skin flap of 3 × 2.5 cm is elevated using an electric dermatome with the site of placement being in the centre of the flap (fig. 3a). To avoid the dermatome to produce an uneven flap, it is important to flatten the area where the local anesthetic has been infiltrated with digital pressure. The SCT is cut out subsequently (fig. 3b). The borders are freed from SCT (fig. 3c) and undermined as described above. The free skin borders are sutured to the periosteum. After placement of the implant (see below), the skin flap is brought back to its original position and sutured, placed directly on the periosteum (fig. 3d). For the exteriorization of the implant, a hole is punched in the flap. This creates a square grove with the screw placed in the centre.

Round Flap (Excised and Reimplanted)
A skin circle 2.5 cm in diameter around the planned site of screw implantation is cut out including

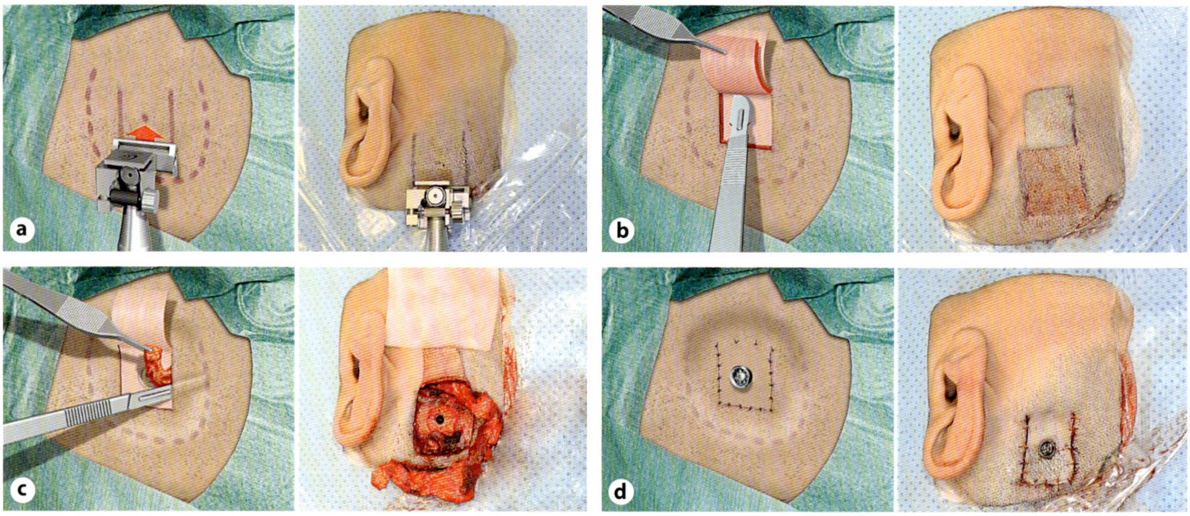

Fig. 3. **a** A square cutaneous skin flap of 3 × 2.5 cm is elevated using an electric dermatome with the site of placement in the centre of the flap. **b** The SCT is resected after development of the skin flap. **c** The borders are freed from SCT and undermined. **d** After placement of the implant, the skin flap is brought back to its original position and sutured, placed directly on the periosteum.

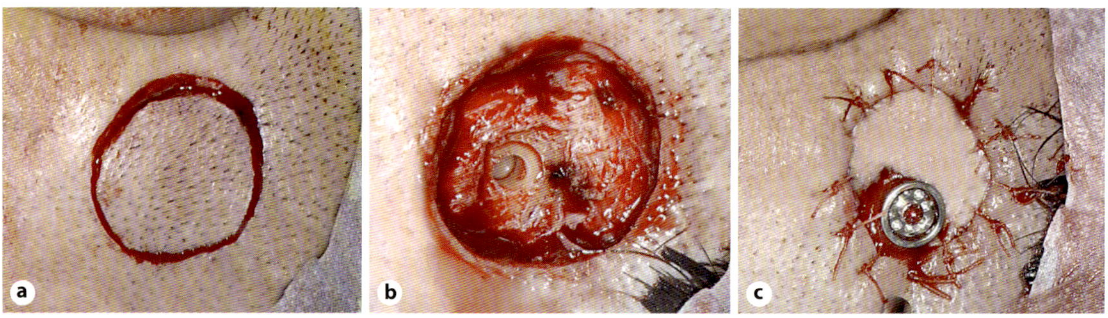

Fig. 4. **a**, **b** For the round flap, a skin circle of 2.5 cm in diameter around the planned site of screw implantation is cut out including the SCT. **c** After placement of the implant, the skin graft is reimplanted and sutured at its original site, placed directly on the periosteum.

the SCT (fig. 4a, b). The borders are freed from SCT and undermined as described above. The free skin borders are sutured to the periosteum. The excised skin is thinned out and therefore cleared from any SCT and hair follicles. After placement of the implant (see below), the skin graft is reimplanted and sutured at its original site, placed directly on the periosteum (fig. 4c). For the exteriorization of the implant, a hole is punched in the flap. This creates a circular grove with the screw placed in the center.

Linear Incision

A straight line incision of about 5 cm is performed with the site of placement in the middle of the incision (fig. 5a). In an area of 25 mm around the

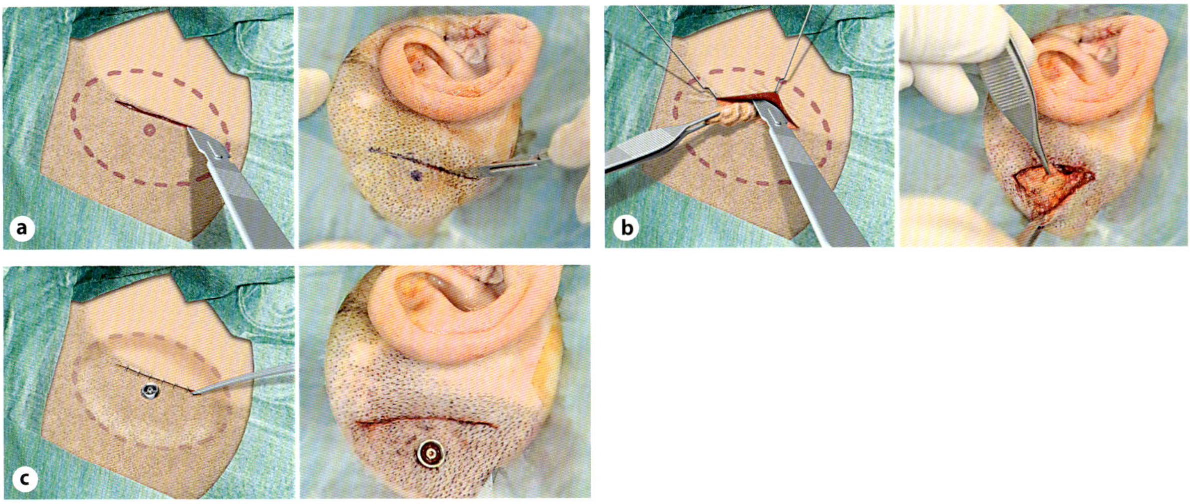

Fig. 5. a A straight line incision of about 5 cm is performed with the site of placement in the middle of the incision. **b** In an area of 25 mm around the place chosen for the implant, the skin borders are undermined and the SCT is resected. **c** After placement of the implant, the skin is sutured down to the periosteum around the implant.

place chosen for the implant, the skin borders are undermined and the SCT is resected (fig. 5b). In the same area, the underside of the skin has to be totally cleared from hair follicles using a fresh blade. After placement of the implant (see below), the skin is sutured down to the periosteum around the implant. This creates a circular grove with the screw placed in the centre (fig. 5c).

Drilling and Insertion of the Titanium Screw

The placement of the screw has to respect the concept of osseointegration.

Osseointegration refers to the fact that the bone and the titanium screw are connected in a direct and fixed manner. This firm integration enables the screw to support high-pressure forces, a fact that is well known from dental implants. Since the introduction of the Baha in 1977, osseointegrated screws are used to transmit vibrations of a bone conduction stimulator to cranial bone and subsequently to the inner ear.

To avoid a bad integration of the screw, several precautions have to be followed. To avoid the implantation of particles from surgical gloves or steel instruments, the titanium screw should not be touched with anything else than the titanium forceps included in the implantation set. All bone preparation must be made without overheating and very slowly in order to avoid carbonization, which is known to impair the process of screw osseointegration. (Osteocytes die after 1 min at 42°C; temperature will reach >100°C when drilling at 2000 rpm.)

The Baha set supplies only two different titanium screws. The only difference is the length of 3 versus 4 mm; according to this the drill can be configured to stop at a depth of 3 or 4 mm. The screw's width is always the same (1.85 mm).

The drilling is performed using a handpiece with a 90° angle from the drill to the bone (fig. 6a). A plastic pointer can be attached to guide the drilling, which has to be exactly perpendicular to the skull bone at the site of implantation. Continuous irrigation with saline solution is important to avoid

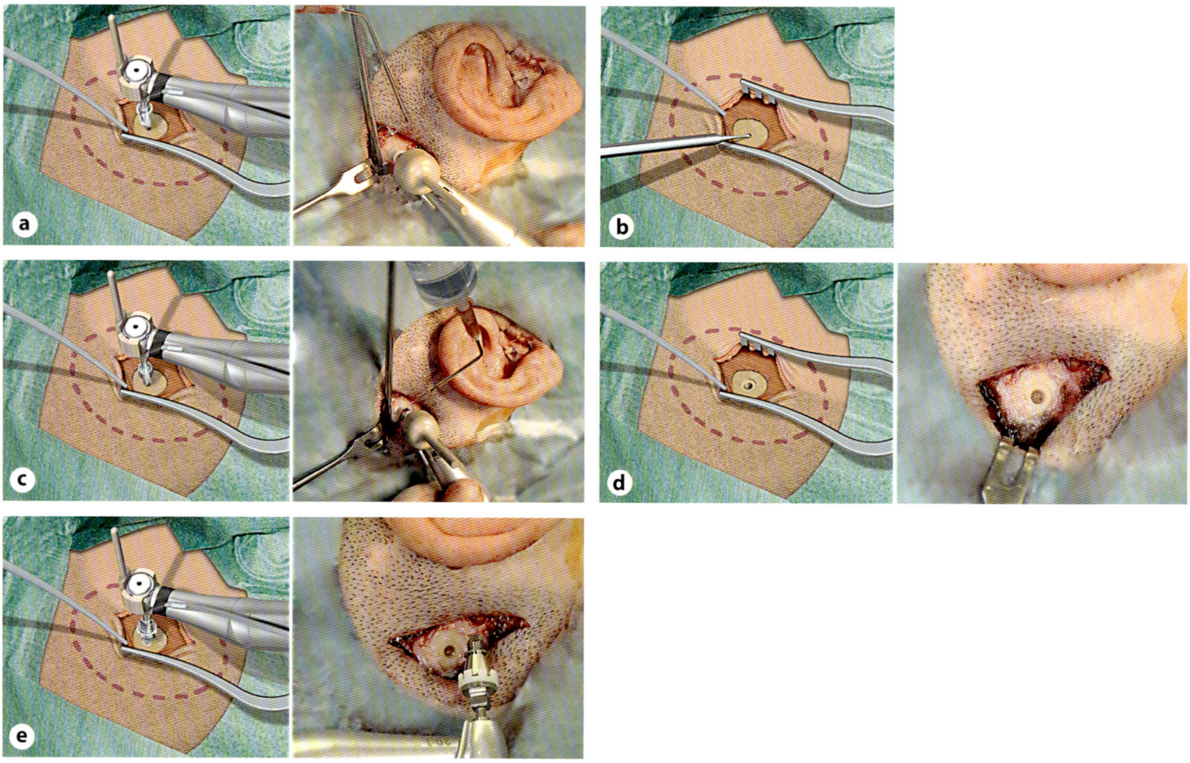

Fig. 6. a The drilling is performed using a handpiece with a 90° angle from the drill to the bone. A plastic pointer can be attached to guide the drilling, which has to be exactly perpendicular to the skull bone at the site of implantation. **b** The bottom of the hole is examined using a small curette, making sure the dura has not already been reached. **c** The width of the hole is enlarged using the countersink. **d** As soon as a slight 'corona' around the hole has been created, the drilling is finished. **e** The screw is inserted in a strict perpendicular way.

overheating. The drill motor is set to the drilling mode. At first, the drill configuration for a depth of 3 mm is used. Subsequently, the bottom of the hole is examined using a small curette, making sure the dura has not already been reached (fig. 6b). If a bony bottom is found, the 4-mm drill is applied. If dura or even cerebrospinal fluid leak is encountered surgical bone wax is used to seal.

Subsequently, the width of the hole is enlarged to 3.50 mm using the countersink of either 3 or 4 mm, according to the hole drilled in the previous step (fig. 6c). The countersink must be moved in and out gently and perpendicular to avoid widening the hole by drilling laterally or at a wrong angle. As soon as a slight 'corona' around the hole has been created, the drilling is finished (fig. 6d).

For the screw placement, the drill motor is set to the screw mode (fixed speed: 15 rpm forward or 30 rpm backward; torque selectable between 10 and 40 Ncm). The screw is inserted in a strict perpendicular way. Again, the use of the pointer can help in this step (fig. 6e).

Wound Closure

After exteriorization of the implanted abutment through a punched hole in the skin flap, the skin borders of the flap are closed while suturing the

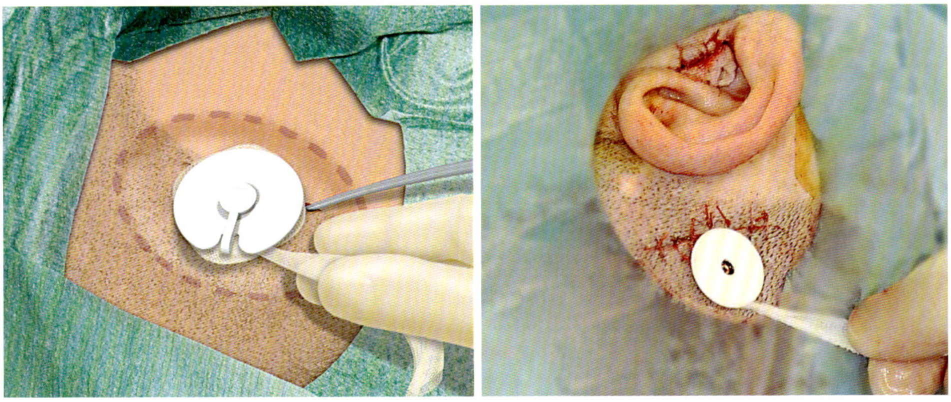

Fig. 7. The healing cap is placed on the abutment. Gauze with ointment containing antibiotics and corticosteroids is rolled up within the cap.

skin borders of the undermined area directly to the periosteum (cf. section 'Alternatives in Skin and Soft Tissue Procedures' above). The healing cap is placed on the abutment. Gauze with ointment containing antibiotics and corticosteroids is rolled up within the cap (fig. 7). This dressing holds the skin in close contact to the underlying skull and avoids the formation of hematoma around the site of implantation. Intensive pressure on the flap should be avoided to prevent tissue necrosis. A circular dressing around the head is usually applied for 24 h.

Alternative: Two-Stage Procedure

In cases of unstable bone, e.g. fibrous dysplasia or osteogenesis imperfecta, a two-stage procedure is indicated. In such a case, the screw is implanted without skin work and placement of the abutment. The implant is left subcutaneously for a prolonged period to assure firm osseointegration (fig. 8). Consequently, a second intervention is performed with preparation of the skin, resection of SCT and placement of the abutment.

Postoperative Care and Follow-Up

The day after surgery, a local wound dressing is applied over the healing cap. The gauze dressing under the healing cap should be changed every week depending on the progress of the healing (from 3 to 6 weeks). After 6–8 weeks, the bone conduction aid can be fitted on the abutment. The patient should be advised to clean the abutment and the implantation site daily with soap water and a soft toothbrush. This is important to prevent irritation by skin debris or even infection. In this context, correct counseling of the patient regarding early signs of possible complications is important.

Conclusion

A good wound healing and no soft tissue overgrowth are the first goals of a successful Baha implantation [4]. The skin around the implant should be thin and without hair follicles [5]. These standardized techniques of Baha implantation have a certain risk of failure. The main complication during the time after implantation is the necrosis of the skin around the implant, which is

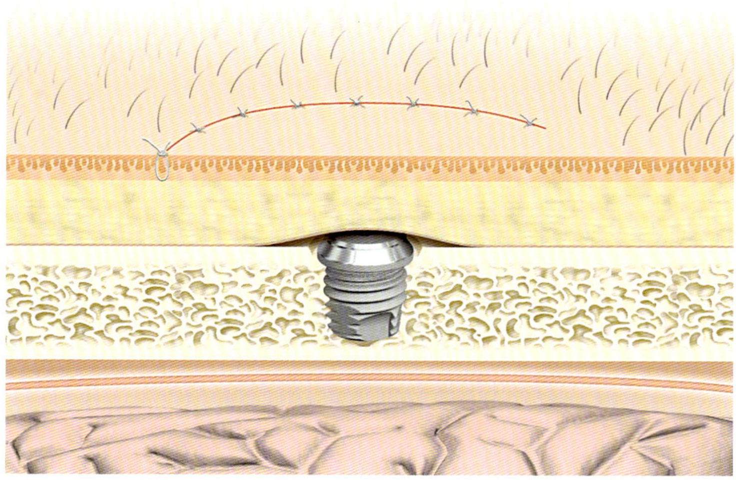

Fig. 8. The implant is left subcutaneously for a prolonged period to assure firm osseointegration.

reported to occur in 1.3–9.6% of cases [6]. There is no statistically significant difference in necrosis of the skin flap between the different techniques [6, 7]. Some authors prefer a specific technique. Recently, the linear incision technique has been advocated, as it is claimed to be easier and with lower incidence of immediate wound problems such as skin necrosis [3, 8]. This has not been statistically proven. But Mudry [3] reported a statistically significant difference in the unscheduled consultations in the skin flap group because of skin irritations and crusting. He assumes the poorer vascularization of the flap is the reason for this finding. Furthermore, a more stable situation is created with the linear incision technique avoiding skin border movements, which could lead to inflammation and tissue overgrowth. According to two studies, there is no difference in the long-term complication rates between the techniques [9, 10].

Thus, if performed carefully, the surgery for the Baha has a favorable outcome, regardless of the technique used.

Acknowledgements

We would like to thank Rom Mendel and Pernilla Petterssion (both Cochlear, Ltd.) for providing illustrations and Aisha Spring for additional artwork.

References

1 Proops DW: Surgery for the bone anchored hearing aid. ENT Audiol News 2010;19:47–49.

2 Wazen JJ, Spitzer JB, Ghossaini SN, et al: Transcranial contralateral cochlear stimulation in unilateral deafness. Otolaryngol Head Neck Surg 2003;129: 248–254.

3 Mudry A: Bone-anchored hearing aids (BAHA): skin healing process for skin flap technique versus linear incision technique in the first three months after the implantation. Rev Laryngol Otol Rhinol (Bord) 2009;130:281–284.

4 Woolford TJ, Morris DP, Saeed SR, Rothera MP: The implant-site split-skin graft technique for the bone-anchored hearing aid. Clin Otolaryngol Allied Sci 1999;24:177–180.

5 Portmann D, Boudard P, Herman D: Anatomical results with titanium implants in the mastoid region. Ear Nose Throat J 1997;76:231–234, 236.
6 Tjellström A, Granström G: How we do it: frequency of skin necrosis after BAHA surgery. Clin Otolaryngol 2006;31: 216–220.
7 Battista RA, Littlefield PD: Revision BAHA surgery. Otolaryngol Clin North Am 2006;39:801–813.
8 de Wolf MJ, Hol MK, Huygen PL, Mylanus EA, Cremers CW: Nijmegen results with application of a bone-anchored hearing aid in children: simplified surgical technique. Ann Otol Rhinol Laryngol 2008;117:805–814.
9 House JW, Kutz JW Jr: Bone-anchored hearing aids: incidence and management of postoperative complications. Otol Neurotol 2007;28: 213–217.
10 de Wolf MJ, Hol MK, Huygen PL, Mylanus EA, Cremers CW: Clinical outcome of the simplified surgical technique for BAHA implantation. Otol Neurotol 2008;29:1100–1108.

Andreas Arnold, MD
Department of ENT, Head and Neck Surgery, Inselspital, University of Bern
CH–3010 Bern (Switzerland)
Tel. +41 31 632 21 11, Fax +41 31 632 49 00, E-Mail andreas.arnold@insel.ch

Kompis M, Caversaccio M-D (eds): Implantable Bone Conduction Hearing Aids.
Adv Otorhinolaryngol. Basel, Karger, 2011, vol 71, pp 56–62

Paediatric Baha

Ann-Louise McDermott[a] · Patrick Sheehan[b]

[a]The Birmingham Children's Hospital, Birmingham, and [b]Royal Manchester Children's Hospital, Manchester, UK

Abstract

Bone-anchored hearing aids (Baha®) are a well-established and readily available option for aural rehabilitation for children. Audiological outcomes and paediatric quality of life results have added to the evidence of benefit of Baha. Recent years have seen an increase in the number of centres worldwide providing a Baha service for children. Indications for Baha have evolved. The paediatric population present a variety of challenges for clinicians who undertake Baha surgery. Complex medical conditions, social and educational issues, and trauma are such examples. The surgical techniques are now varied and the timing of surgery varies between surgeons and Baha centres. Fortunately, serious complications are very rare, and to date there are no more than six significant such case reports in the literature. Careful patient selection and a multidisciplinary team approach with an understanding of the problems that present in children should result in a successful outcome for the child.

The concept of osseointegration and its important role in retention of bone conduction hearing aids has been well established since the bone-anchored hearing aid (Baha®) device became commercially available in 1987 [1]. Today, there are many studies describing both audiological benefits and quality of life outcomes following Baha both in adult and paediatric populations [2–6].

Baha is an accepted form of auditory rehabilitation for adults and children alike. For those clinicians who undertake paediatric Baha practice, the assessment, surgical techniques, complications including trauma present different challenges [7].

In children, general anaesthesia is preferred, and two-staged surgery is often the most appropriate choice. Since many children who require a Baha often have a significant medical and/or syndromic history, the procedure may carry more risk [8].

Soft tissue and skull thickness can vary greatly in young children, and may significantly affect the surgical procedure itself as well as any subsequent complication rates.

Controversy still exists regarding the best time to implant children. The majority of centres are opting to wait until at least 4 years of age. However, the aim is to restore hearing as soon as possible in order for the child to achieve his/her full potential.

Evolving Indications for Baha in Children

Early indications for paediatric Baha were predominantly chronic suppurative otitis media, chronic otitis externa, persistent otitis media with effusion and trauma to the external ear where children could not manage or tolerate conventional hearing aids. Now Baha is the hearing aid of choice for the rehabilitation of children with atretic or microtic ears [7]. The recent role of Baha in unilateral hearing loss, and for children with significant and severe behavioural problems has further expanded the indications [9].

Outcomes from adult Baha users with single-sided deafness have been very positive. These adult patients perceived improvement in directionality of sound particularly in background noise situations [10–12].

Small studies on older children with a single-sided hearing loss did support the adult results; however, young children with congenital unilateral hearing loss were found to have good perception of directionality of sound [13]. Further objective studies on speech in noise did not show any significant improvement after Baha fitting except in those children with a profound unilateral sensorineural hearing loss. Some authors reported noticeable improvements in hearing in noise and in listening difficulties [14, 15].

Overall, there is no convincing evidence for early intervention in those children with unilateral congenital conductive hearing loss providing there is normal hearing in the contralateral ear [16].

When assessing a child with single-sided hearing loss, it is good clinical practice to involve the child's carers in the decision to aid. All children should have a trial of Baha® Softband before a final decision to implant is made.

Similarly, there is increasing evidence that children with severe/profound behavioural difficulties gain significant benefit in quality of life [9].

These children should be considered on an individual basis, and again a fully informed discussion between carers and the multidisciplinary team is recommended before any decision is made for surgery.

Table 1 highlights the most common indications for a Baha in the paediatric population.

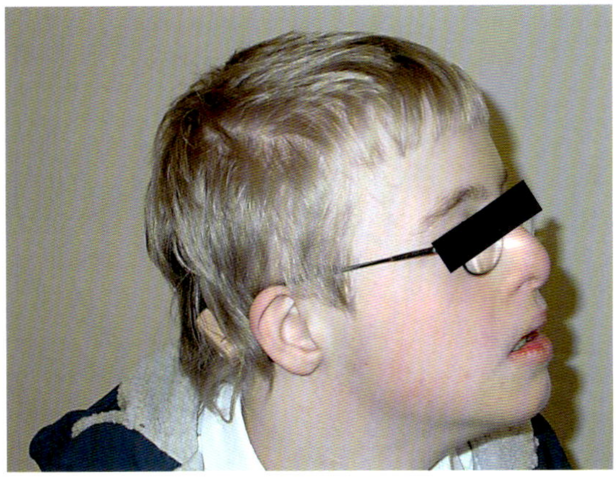

Fig. 1. Young man with Down Syndrome and a Baha.

Table 1. The most common indications for a Baha in the paediatric population

Congenital aural atresia
Congenital microtia
Chronic otitis externa
Persistent otitis media with effusion
Chronic suppurative otitis media
Unilateral profound hearing loss
External ear trauma/burns
Child with conductive/mixed hearing loss unable to tolerate conventional aids

When Is the Best Time to Implant Children?

This question has resulted in much debate. The majority of the paediatric Baha literature suggests waiting until the child is aged 4 years and above.

It had previously been suggested that age 3 years and above is ideal since the child should then have suitable skull thickness [17].

Centres reporting on Baha in very young children highlight a significant increase in perioperative problems with thin calvarial bone and later postoperative complications, particularly fixture loss [18–20]. Children with Treacher Collins and Goldenhar syndromes have been reported to have a higher incidence of bony developmental delay which may influence timing of fixture implantation [18, 21]. Figure 1 shows a young man with Down syndrome who has managed well with his Baha.

The use of the Baha on a test band is considered the gold standard for audiological preoperative assessment in children, but importantly the Baha Softband provides aural rehabilitation to very young children who are not yet at an appropriate age for surgery [22].

Management of older children with a Baha headband may be more challenging. Self-image and peer pressure surrounding the appearance of the test bands may result in poor compliance despite good audiological outcomes. This is more of a problem in boys who may have shorter hair styles. Similar problems are not uncommon in children with learning difficulties who may have issues tolerating the headband.

The authors of this article recommend the use of the Baha Softband until age 4 years. This practice allows for customisation and tolerance of the Baha.

There are studies reporting successful implantation in under 3-year-olds; however, other factors such as prolonged osseointegration times are practiced [23].

Two-stage surgery is standard practice for children. It allows the very important undisturbed osseointegration period to occur.

There are few reports of single-stage surgery in young children [24, 25], although it is reported that a one-stage procedure is successful if a 4-mm fixture is used [1].

Sheehan and Rothera [26] have described a modified two-stage procedure suitable for older children. The soft tissue stages are carried out at the time of the initial fixture placement. Once sufficient osseointegration time has passed, the previously prepared skin graft is punctured under local anaesthetic and the abutment attached in the outpatient (office) setting. This has the advantage of not requiring a second general anaesthetic.

Recent reports describe modifications of Baha surgical techniques [27]. Recent years have seen the introduction of the Baha® Dermatome. This gives reproducible results with the thin split thickness graft [28].

Recent linear incision technique described by the Nijmegen team [19] is reported to have fewer complications and is gaining in popularity. This linear incision does not require a skin graft but emphasises the importance of undermining the surrounding skin. There are others who report a simplified technique without a skin flap, again with few complications but their study numbers have been small and it is not yet performed on children [29].

Caution is advised when considering Baha in children with congenital abnormalities of the external ear. The abnormal anatomy may be misleading when deciding fixture placement. Furthermore, if autologous reconstruction is to be considered at a later stage, then posterior placement is recommended to avoid compromising the healthy tissues at the site of the future surgery [30].

The use of a sleeper fixture (spare fixture) is recommended in children, especially those below the age of 10 years due to the increased rates of fixture failure and trauma. It is commonly an ipsilateral fixture close to the primary fixture.

There is some evidence that there is an increased fixture failure rate with the shorter fixtures [20]. It has been suggested that 2 mm of cortical bone thickness is necessary for implantation for a Baha [23]. The Nijmegen team interestingly did not find the age or fixture length to influence fixture stability [19]. Davids [23] described the placement of a 3-mm fixture flush with the outer bone table (dura depressed by the fixture), then a longer period of healing time before stage II. The author found this reduced the need for multiple pilot holes. Studies from the Birmingham team reported few complications with the predominant use of 3-mm fixtures [21].

Fixture failure rates of children below the age of 5 years and those 5–10 years are 40 and 8%, respectively. Those children over the age of 10 years have 1% fixture loss [18, 21, 31]. Recent suggestions have been to place the sleeper fixture on the contralateral side in bilateral cases, thus reducing the overall costs and allowing the option of bilateral Baha use [32].

Fixture stability is affected by a combination of factors such as trauma and skin reactions around the abutment. However, the majority of fixture failures are spontaneous and the cause remains unclear.

At the time of surgery, inadequate bone thickness can be managed by using a Gortex augmentation technique, which has been well described [33]. Another alternative is to collect the bone dust/chips from the countersink and pack them around the fixture flange.

The ideal time between fixture implantation and placing the abutment (osseointegration time) continues to be a topic of debate. A 3-month period between surgeries has been common practice in the majority of paediatric Baha centres. If difficulties are encountered at the first procedure such as inadequate bone thickness, a longer osseointegration period is recommended. Authors describing the use of a 4-mm fixture in all cases irrespective of bone thickness have reported osseointegration times in excess of 6 months [1, 23]. Newer implant fixtures BI300 have been designed to increase the tissue response and thus reduce the osseointegration time period before the sound processor can be fitted. The early results have been very positive in animal models and the adequate osseointegration remains to be seen in adults and children [34].

Complications

Increased complication rates following paediatric Baha surgery are well recognised compared to adult Baha series [1, 18, 21, 23, 35–37].

Loss of the fixture due to failure of osseointegration is significantly higher in younger children [19, 21]. There is a general consensus that fixture failure is most common in the first postoperative year [19].

Soft tissue complications are the most common problem encountered.

The responsibility for cleaning and care of the percutaneous abutment and surrounding soft tissues falls in most cases to the child's carers.

The hygiene of the family/older child/carer should be taken into account when deciding to proceed with a Baha.

For those children with challenging behaviour, cleaning of the abutment may prove to be more demanding. Significant hypertrophy of the skin surrounding the abutment may require skin reduction. Recent reports describe a topical steroid gel (clobetasol 0.05%) applied to the skin surrounding the abutment to be beneficial, but caution must be exercised when using steroids in children [38].

Older children are at risk of sebaceous gland hypertrophy and acne [39]. Any resulting skin overgrowth may be dealt with by changing to a longer (8.5 mm) abutment [40].

The pathogenesis of the soft tissue complications is believed to result from a foreign body reaction to keratin and keratinocytes at the titanium/bone interface [41].

Trauma to the Baha is a challenge to any centre providing a paediatric BAHA service. Fortunately, this is usually damage to the Baha sound processor, but abutment damage can occur. The

Table 2. Unusual serious complications with the use of a BAHA

Year	Age	Complication	First author
1993	adult	intracerebral abscess	Dietmer [43]
2003	child	intracranial intrusion of fixture	Dietmer [43]
2003	42 years	intracranial abscess	Scholz [44]
2003	68 years	bronchogenic metastasis to Baha site	Hadjihannas [45]
2008	9 years	intracranial intrusion of fixture	McDermott [42]
2010	15 years	epidural haematoma	Mestfin [46]

incidence of significant complications resulting from trauma to the Baha fixture/abutment remains very low. Unexpected and unusual complications can occur long after the Baha surgery [42] (table 2).

Paediatric quality of life studies following the provision of a Baha have been reported by most Baha centres [2–4, 7, 14, 17–19, 21, 22, 48–50].

The overwhelming finding from all these studies is the significant improvement in hearing rehabilitation and quality of life in children using Baha.

Finally, recent literature reports success rates of 96% and above in all the large paediatric Baha centres. Success has been determined by the number of hours per day each week that the child wore the Baha [16, 18, 19, 21, 36, 41, 47–51].

Conclusions

The Baha system has been proven to be a success in rehabilitating the hearing loss in children with conductive hearing loss who are unable to wear conventional hearing aids for particular reasons. The Baha surgery in children is different to surgery in adults with unique challenges related to implanting children particularly those with other co-morbidities or those children with learning difficulties. However, the results are encouraging in children with clear evidence of improved quality of life for these children. A multidisciplinary team approach with careful patient selection has improved the outcome of paediatric Baha surgery. Newer technologies and evolving surgical techniques are continually improving benefits of Baha surgery.

References

1 Tietze L, Papsin B: Utilization of bone-anchored hearing aids in children. Int J Pediatr Otorhinolaryngol 2001;58:75–80.

2 Mylanus EAM, Snik AFM, Cremers CWRJ: Patients' opinions of bone-anchored vs conventional hearing aids. Arch Otolaryngol Head Neck Surg 1995;121:421–425.

3 Dutt SN, McDermott AL, Jelbert A, Reid AP, Proops DW: The Glasgow Benefit Inventory in the evaluation of patient satisfaction with the bone-anchored hearing aid: quality of life issues. J Laryngol Otol Supp 2002;28:7–14.

4 Hol MKS, Spath MA, Krabbe PFM, van der Pouw CTM, Snik AFM, Cremers CWRJ, Mylanus EAM: The bone-anchored hearing aid: quality-of-life assessment. Arch Otolaryngol Head Neck Surg 2004;130:394–399.

5 Gillett D, Fairley JW, Chandrashake RTS, Bean A, Gonzalez J: Bone-anchored hearing aids: results of the first eight years of a programme in a district general hospital, assessed by the Glasgow Benefit Inventory. J Laryngol Otol 2006;120:537–542.
6 Saliba I, Woods O, Caron C: BAHA results in children at one year follow-up: a prospective longitudinal study. Int J Pediatr Otorhinolaryngol 2010;74: 1058–1062.
7 McDermott AL, Sheehan P: Bone anchored hearing aids in children. Curr Opin Otolaryngol head Neck Surg 2009;17:488–493.
8 Stevenson DS, Proops DW, Wake MJC, Deadman MJ, Worollo SJ: Osseointegrated implants in the management of childhood ear abnormalities: the initial Birmingham experience. J Laryngol Otol 1993;107:502–509.
9 Doshi J, McDermott AL, Reid A, Proops D: The use of a bone-anchored hearing aid (Baha) in children with severe behavioural problems – the Birmingham Baha programme experience. Int J Pediatr Otorhinolaryngol 2010;74:608–610.
10 Wazen JJ, Spitzer J, Ghossaini SN: Results of the bone anchored hearing aid in unilateral hearing loss. Laryngoscope 2001;111:955–958.
11 Snik AFM, Mylanus EAM, Cremers CWRJ: The bone anchored hearing aid in patients with a unilateral air-bone gap. Otol Neurotol 2002;23:61–66.
12 Linstrom CJ, Silverman CA, Yu GP: Efficacy of the bone anchored hearing aid for single sided deafness. Laryngoscope 2009;119:713–720.
13 Christensen L, Dornhoffer JL: Bone anchored hearing aids for unilateral hearing loss in teenagers. Otol Neurotol 2008;29:1120–1122.
14 Kunst SJW, Leijendeckers JM, Mylanus EAM, Hol MKS, Snik AFM, Cremers CWRJ: BAHA system application for unilateral congenital conductive hearing impairment: audiometric results. Otol Neurotol 2008;29:2–7.
15 Christensen L, Richter GT, Dornhoffer JL: Update on bone-anchored hearing aids in pediatric patients with profound unilateral sensorineural hearing loss. Arch Otolaryngol Head Neck Surg 2010; 136:175–177.
16 Snik AFM, Leijendeckers J, Hol MKS, Mylanus EAM, Cremers CWRJ: The bone anchored hearing aid for children: recent developments. Int J Audiol 2008; 47:554–559.
17 Tjellstrom A, Hakansson B, Granstrom G: Bone anchored hearing aids: current status in adults and children. Otolaryngol Clin North Am 2001;34:337–364.
18 Lloyd S, Almedya J, Sirimanna KS, Albert DM, Bailey CM: Updated surgical experience with bone anchored hearing aids in children. J Laryngol Otol 2007; 121:826–831.
19 De Wolf MJ, Hol MK, Huygen PL, Mylanus EAM, Cremers CW: Nijmegen results with application of a bone anchored hearing aid in children: simplified surgical technique. Ann Otol Rhino Laryngol 2008;117:805–814.
20 Granstrom G, Bergstrom K, Odersjo M, Tjellstrom A: Osseointegrated implants in children: experience from our first 100 patients. Otolaryngol Head Neck Surg 2001;125:85–92.
21 McDermott AL, Williams J, Kuo MJ, Reid AP, Proops DW: The Birmingham Paediatric Bone Anchored Hearing programme: a 15 year experience. Otol Neurotol 2009;30:173–183.
22 Hol MKS, Cremers CWRJ, Coppens-Schellekens W, Snik AFM: The BAHA Softband. A new treatment for young children with bilateral congenital aural atresia. Int J Pediatr Otorhinolaryngol 2005;69:973–980.
23 Davids T: Bone anchored hearing aids in infants and children younger than 5 years. Arch Otolaryngol Head Neck Surg 2007;133:51–55.
24 Kohan D, Morris LG, Romo T: Single stage implantation in adults and children: is it safe? Otolaryngol Head Neck Surg 2008;138:662–666.
25 Ali S, Hadoura L, Carmichael A, Geddes NK: Bone-anchored hearing aid. A single-stage procedure in children. Int J Pediatr Otorhinolaryngol 2009;73: 1076–1079.
26 Sheehan PZ, Rothera M: Two-stage BAHA with one general anaesthetic in children. Clin Otolaryngol 2009;34: 269–270.
27 van de Berg R, Stokroos RJ, Hof JR, Chenault MN: Bone-anchored hearing aid: a comparison of surgical techniques. Otol Neurotol 2010;31:129–135.
28 Stalfors J, Tjellstrom A: Skin reactions after Baha surgery: a comparison between the U-graft technique and the BAHA dermatome. Otol Neurotol 2008; 29:1109–1114.
29 Bovo R: Simplified technique without skin flap for the bone anchored hearing aid implant. Acta Otorhinolaryngol 2008;28:252–255.
30 Proops DW, Wake MJC, Deadman MJ, Worollo SJ: Osseointegrated implants in the management of childhood ear abnormalities: the initial Birmingham experience. J Laryngol Otol 1993;107: 502–509.
31 McDermott AL, Williams J, Kuo MJ, Reid AP, Proops DW: Bone anchored hearing aids in very young children, personal commun.
32 Bernstein JM, Sheehan PZ: An approach to bilateral bone anchored hearing aid surgery in children: contralateral placement of sleeper fixture. J Laryngol Otol 2009;123:555–557.
33 Tjellstrom A, Lindstrom J, Hallen O, Albrektsson T, Branemark P: Osseointegrated titanium implants in the temporal bone. Am J Otol 1981;2:304–310.
34 Gottlow J, Sennerby L, Rosengren A, Flynn M: An experimental evaluation of a new craniofacial implant using the rabbit tibia model. I. Histologic findings. Otol Neurotol 2010;31:832–839.
35 Tjellstrom A, Lindstrom J, Hallen O, Albrektsson T, Branemark P: Osseointegrated titanium implants in the temporal bone. Am J Otol 1981;2:304–310.
36 Sheehan PZ, Hans PS: UK and Ireland experience of bone anchored hearing aids (Baha) in individuals with Down syndrome. Int J Pediatr Otorhinolaryngol 2006;70:981–986.
37 McDermott, Williams J, Kuo MJ, Reid AP, Proops DW: The role of bone anchored hearing aids in children with Down syndrome. Int J Pediatr Otorhinolaryngol 2008;72:751–757.
38 Falcone MT, Kaylie DM, Labadie RF, Haynes DS: Bone anchored hearing aid abutment skin overgrowth reduction with clobetasol. Otolaryngol Head Neck Surg 2008;139:829–832.
39 Priwin C, Granstrom G: The bone anchored hearing aid in children; a surgical and questionnaire follow up study. Otolaryngol Head Neck Surg 2005;132: 559–565.

40 Monksfield P, Ho EC, Reid AP, Proops DW: Experience with the longer (8.5 mm) abutment for bone anchored hearing aid. Otol Neurotol 2009;30:274–276.
41 Khwaja S, Curry A, Chaudhry IH, Green KM: Can keratinocytes cause failure of osseointegration? J Laryngol Otol 2009; 123:1035–1038.
42 McDermott AL, Barraclough J, Reid AP: Trauma, unusual complications and findings with bone anchored hearing aids: report of a case and review of the literature. J Laryngol Otol 2009;123: 348–350.
43 Dietmer T, Krassort M, Hartmann S: Two rare complications in patients with bone anchored hearing aids (in German). Laryngorhinootologie 2003;82: 162–165.
44 Scholz M, Eufinger H, Anders A, Illerhaus B, Matthias K, Schmieder K, Harders A: Intra-cerebral abscess after abutment change of a bone anchored hearing aid. Otol Neurotol 2003;24:896–899.
45 Hadjihannas E, McDermott AL, Warfield AT, Proops DW, Reid AP: Occult bronchogenic carcinoma presenting as metastasis to the site of a Bone anchored hearing aid. J Laryngol Otol 2003;117: 396–398.
46 Mestfin FB, Perkins NW, Brook C, Foyt D, German JW: Epidural hematoma after tympanomastoidectomy and bone anchored hearing aid placement. Neurosurgery 2010;65:E1451–E1453.
47 Kunst SJW, Hol MKS, Cremers CWRJ, Mylanus EAM: The bone anchored hearing aid in patients with moderate mental retardation: impact and benefit assessment. Otol Neurotol 2007;28:793–797.
48 Dun CA, de Wolf MJ, Mylanus EA, Snik AF, Hol MK, Cremers CW: Bilateral bone-anchored hearing aid application in children: the Nijmegen experience from 1996 to 2008. Otol Neurotol 2010;31:615–623.
49 Ricci G, Della Volpe A, Faralli M, Longari F, Gullà M, Mansi N, Frenguelli A: Results and complications of the Baha system (bone-anchored hearing aid). Eur Arch Otorhinolaryngol 2010;267:1539–1545.
50 McDermott AL, Williams J, Kuo MJ, et al: Quality of life in children fitted with a bone anchored hearing aid. Otol Neurotol 2009;30:344–349.
51 Tjellstrom A: Osseointegrated implants for the replacement of absent or defected ears. Clin Plast Surg 1990;17:355–366.

Miss Ann-Louise McDermott
Department of Otolaryngology, The Birmingham Children's Hospital
Steelhouse Lane
Birmingham B4 6NH (UK)
Tel. +44 121 333 8123, Fax +44 121 333 8121, E-Mail annlouise.mcdermott@bch.nhs.uk

Kompis M, Caversaccio M-D (eds): Implantable Bone Conduction Hearing Aids.
Adv Otorhinolaryngol. Basel, Karger, 2011, vol 71, pp 63–72

Complications of Bone-Anchored Hearing Devices

Jack J. Wazen · Benjamin Wycherly · Julie Daugherty

Silverstein Institute, Ear Research Foundation, Sarasota, Fla., USA

Abstract

Complications of bone-anchored hearing devices occur with both soft tissue and bone. Soft tissue complications are much more common and most often involve irritation of the skin surrounding the implant. Other complications include: skin flap necrosis, wound dehiscence, bleeding or hematoma formation, and persistent pain. Bone complications are classified as either early or late. Early complications are due to failure of osseointegration, while late complications are usually the result of either chronic infection or trauma. Pediatric patients are a unique group of implant patients and are more likely to have complications of both soft tissue and bone. Most complications can be managed in the office with topical therapy and wound care, although revision surgery may be required in extensive skin overgrowth cases. Proper patient selection, meticulous surgical technique, and patient hygiene around the implant are the most critical aspects in minimizing complications in patients with osseointegrated implants.

The principles of osseointegration and the surgical techniques have been covered elsewhere and will not be repeated in this chapter. Our focus here will be on the complications encountered in such surgery, how to treat them and how to avoid them. We will divide the complications into bone and soft tissue complications, and include a discussion of pediatric considerations.

The simplicity, high success rate and patient satisfaction in the osseointegrated auditory implants far outweigh the surgical risks and complications. However, failure to adhere to the basic surgical principles of the procedure has led to higher reported complication rates in some centers and patient populations. We will therefore describe the different types of complications and how to avoid them.

Bone Complications

Implant Loss

Complications related to the bone causing implant loss can be categorized as early (failure of osseointegration) or delayed (loss of osseointegration, or 'disintegration') [1].

Prerequisites for successful osseointegration include: status of bone, implant design, implant material and finish, surgical technique and implant loading conditions [2].

Numerous studies report various rates of bone complications and implant loss for bone-anchored hearing aid (Baha) recipients. Early failure of osseointegration resulting in implant loss ranged from 0.4 to 9.3% [3–5], while delayed implant loss caused by infection or trauma ranged from 0.4 to 2.7% [6–10]. Children have a higher rate of implant loss [11]. Faber et al. [12] propose the cause of the higher extrusion rate in children is that the child's skull is thinner and has a lower mineral content compared to the adult skull. Skull thickness is not just dependent on age, but also related to craniofacial abnormalities such as in Treacher-Collins' syndrome [13]. Reyes et al. [6] suggest that bone resorption at the bone-metal surface causes implant loss when there is no history of trauma. Implant loss rates in children range from 5.3 to 30%, with a greater proportion reported as early failures [14–17]. In a series of children implanted under the age of 5 years at The Birmingham BAHA program, an implant failure rate of 40% was reported [11]. Infection, incomplete implant insertion, failure of osseointegration and trauma have been reported as the main causes of implant loss in the pediatric population [13]. The evolution of the surgical technique to include placement of a spare implant (sleeper) in children during the initial surgery has reduced the rate of replacement surgery [3]. However, factors that contribute to loss of the primary implant may affect the integrity of the sleeper [13].

The implant size indicated for the pediatric population has been disputed by clinicians. Some studies report an increased implant loss rate with 3-mm implants [16, 18–19]. However, de Wolf et al. [3] and Lloyd et al. [14] found no significant difference in implant length and rate of implant loss. Further, they found no correlation between osseointegration in drill holes that ended in bone and those which exposed dura or the sigmoid sinus. Current evidence confirms the minimal temporal bone thickness needed to hold a 3-mm implant is 2.5 mm [20].

Other population subsets that have been identified to have an increased incidence of bone complications include patients with diabetes mellitus, chronic steroid use and smokers [21–24]. Animal studies have established that diabetes impedes osseointegration of titanium implants [25]. Studies show patients with pre-existing conditions that affect wound healing and bone density need longer than 3 months for complete osseointegration, and delayed loading with the processor to reduce the risk of implant extrusion [26]. No studies are available evaluating osseointegration in bone diseases. However, Uppal et al. [27] report successful Baha surgery and sustained osseointegration of an implant in a 72-year-old man with advanced Paget's disease. Studies demonstrate that bone complications do not increase in the elderly population that is predisposed to diseases that diminish bone density, such as osteoporosis [18].

Another group that demonstrate a higher bone complication rate are patients who have undergone radiation therapy to the implant region. Ganström [28] found that the adjunctive use of hyperbaric oxygen therapy enhances osseointegration. In these patients and those with pre-existing bone disease, the two-stage technique is recommended.

Clinical standards of care to promote osseointegration in Baha surgery include [18]:

- proper selection of the implant site, preferably along the temporalis line where the bone is thicker with smaller air cells
- fastidious surgical technique with constant cooling irrigation of the implant site and proper handling of the implant
- uninterrupted connection between bone and implant
- adequate healing time
- even distribution of stress over the implant

Bone Infection

The incidence of osteitis is quite rare, and even in cases of recurrent soft tissue infections, the bone appears to be quite resistant to infection. Only one case of an intracranial complication from a Baha has been reported in the literature [29]. This occurred after an unsuccessful attempt at changing the abutment and was subsequently complicated by prolonged postoperative wound infection that developed into an intracerebral abscess.

Soft Tissue Complications

Complications of Baha most commonly involve the soft tissue surrounding the implant. The goal of soft tissue handling in Baha surgery is decreased mobility of soft tissue relative to bone, hairless skin, and a gentle slope of the soft tissue toward the implant. Immobile skin reduces inflammation and the occurrence of skin hypertrophy or scarring. Hair removal decreases skin reactions and allows for improved postoperative hygiene around the abutment. Soft tissue reduction reduces the accumulation of epithelial debris trapped between the abutment and the skin. Although implantation itself is relatively straightforward, attention to detail and delicate soft tissue handling minimizes soft tissue complications.

Intraoperative Complications

Intraoperative complications are rare. The most common issue that arises intraoperatively is bleeding from the scalp, emissary veins, as well as the temporalis and sternocleidomastoid muscles. Bleeding should be controlled with bipolar electrocautery to avoid excessive injury to the blood supply of the thinned skin flap. Exposure of the sigmoid sinus or dura mater may also occur but rarely results in complications. Inadvertent penetration of the transverse or sigmoid sinus occurs rarely and can be controlled easily by inserting bone wax or muscle and redrilling at a nearby site [5, 18].

Postoperative Complications

Bleeding

Persistent postoperative bleeding or the occurrence of a hematoma is rare. Wazen et al. [1] reported 1 case of postoperative bleeding and 1 case of a hematoma formation in 223 implants. de Wolf et al. [30] reported no cases of persistent bleeding and 1 case of a hematoma in 248 implants. In the Hobson et al. [31] review of 602 implants, only 2 patients had persistent bleeding, and 1 patient developed a hematoma after surgery. Hematomas need to be evacuated promptly to avoid flap necrosis from devascularization.

Flap Necrosis

Flap or skin graft necrosis may occur in 0–10% of patients, and usually occurs at areas with inadequate blood supply [3] (fig. 1). Other rare causes of necrosis include excessive pressure over the flap. Tjellstrom and Granstrom [32] reported the incidence of partial and total necrosis of free skin grafts or pedicled skin grafts. The occurrence of partial necrosis and total necrosis in a hairless skin graft was 15.7 and 0.9%. A pedicled skin graft fashioned with a scalpel decreased the rates to 9.8 and 0.6%. The introduction and use of the electric dermatome in 2001 reduced the incidence further to 3 and 0% (fig. 2) [32]. It has been reported recently that the use of a single incision can nearly eliminate flap necrosis. De Wolf et al. [3] reported no flap necrosis in 224 implants using the single incision technique, while Mudry [33] had 1 case of partial necrosis out of 51 implantations. Elimination of flap necrosis can be realized with gentle soft tissue handling, minimum use of cautery, gentle postoperative packing or the use of a single incision (fig. 3).

Partial flap necrosis is successfully managed with appropriate local wound care. Granulation tissue should be treated with silver nitrate with debridement of any devitalized skin.

Skin Irritation and Infection

Postoperative skin inflammation and infection around the abutment is by far the most common complication in Baha surgery. Several large studies have been recently published which review

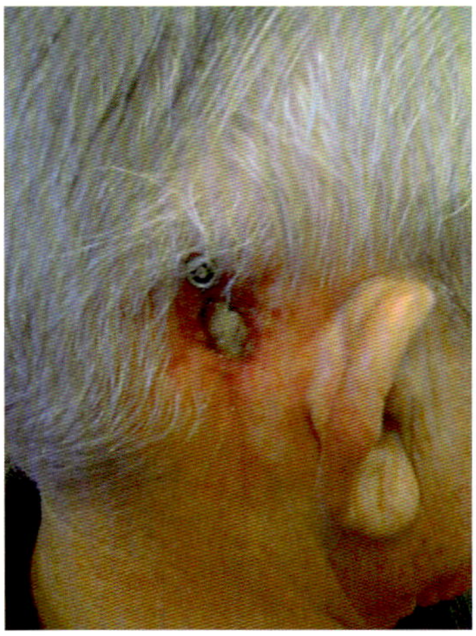

Fig. 1. Partial flap necrosis.

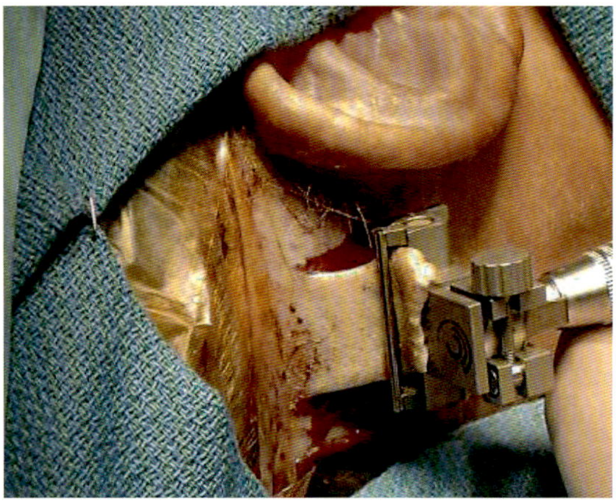

Fig. 2. Flap raising with dermatome.

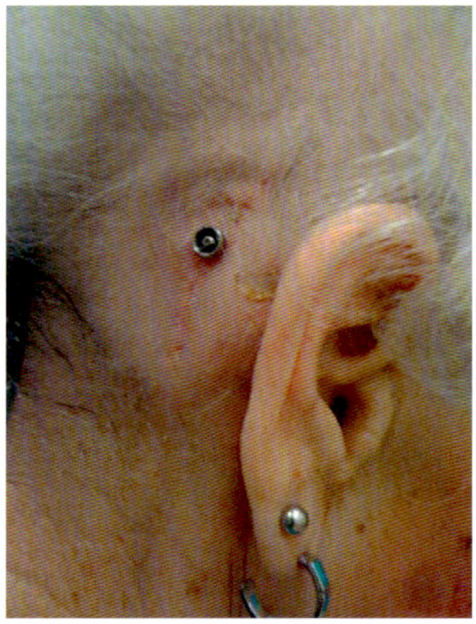

Fig. 3. Single incision.

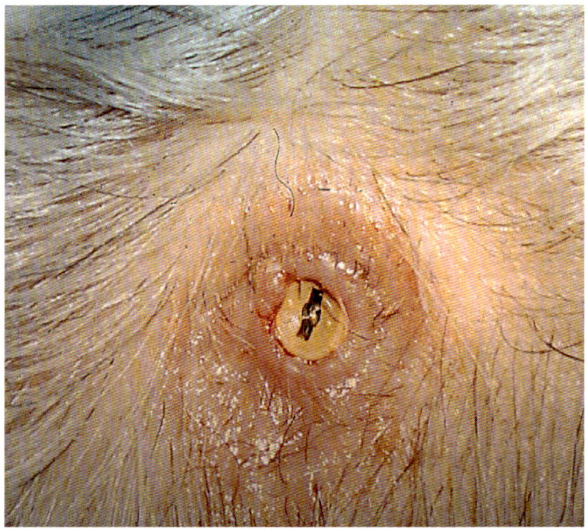

Fig. 4. Hypertrophic skin reaction. Modified Holgers 5.

soft tissue complications, including the incidence of skin reactions after implantation (table 1). The Holgers grading system of postoperative skin irritation was published in 1988 (table 2) [34]. A modification of this grading system was proposed in 2008 by the senior author in order to distinguish between patients successfully treated in the office without the need for revision surgery from those who do require revision surgery (table 3; fig. 4) [1].

Skin reactions around the implant should be avoided because they can result in skin overgrowth, failure of integration, extrusion, and severe wound infection. Fortunately the majority of skin reactions are a Holgers grade 1 (table 4), which almost invariably responds to topical therapy with an

Table 1. Incidence of soft tissue complications

First author	Year	Implants	Observations or years F/U	Age years	Incidence of soft tissue	Incidence of bone	Surgical revision rate	Surgical method
House [8]	2007	149	NR	2–85	9.4% patients	3.4% patients	10%	pedicled flap (dermatome)
Wazen [1]	2008	223	3.7 years	6–92	13% implants	1.3% implants	5.8%	FTSG, pedicled flap
de Wolf [30]	2009	248	1,180 obs.	60–87	12.3% F/U visits	6.5% implants	2.4%	linear incision
Faber [12]	2009	248	1,777 obs.	>17	15.3% F/U visits	1.3% implants	NR	linear incision
Hobson [31]	2010	602	≥1 year	4–87	18.1% implants	4.9% implants	12.1%	STSG

F/U = Follow-up; FTSG = full-thickness skin graft; STSG = split-thickness skin graft; NR = not reported.

Table 2. Holgers classification [34]

Grade 0	No irritation
Grade 1	Slight redness
Grade 2	Red and moist tissue
Grade 3	Granulation tissue
Grade 4	Infection leading to removal of the abutment

antimicrobial/steroid ointment. Granulation tissue should be treated with silver nitrate as well as topical antibiotics, and more significant infections (grade 2–4) may require oral antibiotics. Prompt treatment is paramount. If inflammation or infection is not treated promptly, the integrity of the implant is at stake. House and Kutz [8] reported implant extrusions in 5 patients (3.4%), with 4 of the 5 patients having local inflammation around the implant suggestive of an infection as the cause of integration failure. All occurred between 1 and 4 months after surgery. Patients should be followed closely, especially during the first few months

Table 3. Modified grading system (Wazen) [1]

Grade 0	No irritation: epithelial debris removed if present
Grade 1	Slight redness: temporary local treatment indicated
Grade 2	Red and slightly moist; no granulation tissue present
Grade 3	Red and moist with granulation tissue, skin overgrowth, or scar formation: local treatment indicated
Grade 4	Extensive granulation, skin overgrowth, or scar formation requiring revision surgery
Grade 5	Removal of skin-penetrating abutment necessary to control infection

Table 4. Frequency of Holgers grade 0–4

Study	Holgers grade	Observations
Faber [12]	0	1,505 (84.7%)
	1	206 (11.6%)
	2	52 (2.9%)
	3	12 (0.7%)
	4	2 (0.1%)

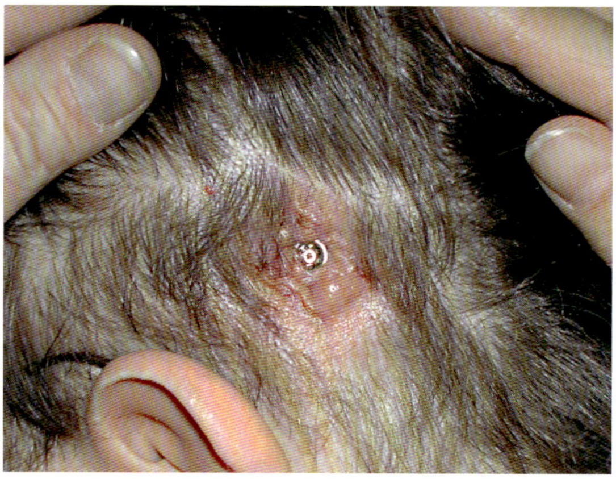

Fig. 5. Keloid formation.

after implantation to assess for skin reactions, and should be advised to maintain a low threshold for follow-up if pain or irritation ensues.

Skin Overgrowth
In our reported series of 223 implants, 4 patients (1.8%) had skin overgrowth and granulation tissue excised in the office, and 10 (4.5%) needed more formal excision and flap revision in the operating room [1]. Patients with inadequate soft tissue thinning, especially if overweight with a thick scalp, are more likely to develop soft tissue overgrowth requiring revision surgery. In a review of 602 patients, Hobson et al. [31] reported soft tissue overgrowth in 48 (8%) of implants, 38 (6%) of which required revision surgery. In an effort to avoid revision surgery, Falcone et al. (2008) reported their use of the superpotent topical steroid clobetasol. Of 13 patients treated with clobetasol, 11 (85%) had resolution of tissue overgrowth without the need for revision surgery [35]. Intralesional steroid injections may help reduce skin overgrowth and avoid revision surgery (fig. 5).

Pain and Paresthesias
Patients are informed about the expected numbness at the surgical site. The area of numbness shrinks over 4–6 months to a small remnant, if any. As many as 4% of patients will have persistent pain at the implant site and may require explantation after Baha surgery [1, 18]. Out of 500 implants, Mylanus et al. [36] reported the removal of 10 (2%) due to persistent pain despite conservative treatment and removal of the abutment. Seven of the implants were evaluated histologically, but were found to be unrevealing in both the soft tissue and the bone. Explantation eliminated the pain in 5 implants, was diminished in 1, and 1 patient reported no change [36]. Despite the inability to explain the cause of persistent pain at the implant site, it is good to inform all patients of the possibility of temporary numbness and persistent pain around the implant, which may require eventual explantation.

Pediatric Patients and Soft Tissue Complications

Baha in children is associated with a higher incidence of soft tissue and bone complications (table 5). This higher incidence of skin reactions is probably because children are more susceptible to trauma, are less likely to maintain adequate hygiene around the abutment, have more reactive skin, have an increased number of active sebaceous glands, and have the propensity to develop soft tissue and bony hypertrophy [6]. Thickening of subcutaneous tissue around the implant in pediatric patients has been noted to be more apparent around puberty [5]. Additionally, many pediatric patients implanted with a Baha are syndromic. This creates additional challenges related to adequate hygiene and trauma to the implant. Many authors have stressed the need for good patient selection, education, and involvement of the caregiver when considering Baha in children. Despite these concerns, there are several studies which indicate that syndromic patients or patients with severe behavioral problems do not have a higher soft tissue complication rate over other children [37, 38].

Table 5. Soft tissue complication rates in the pediatric population

First author	Year	Implants	Observations or years F/U	Age years	Incidence of soft tissue	Incidence of bone	Surgical revision rate	Surgical method
Granstöm [15]	2001	100[1] (76 Baha)	1,140 obs.	≤16	9.1% obs.	5.8% implants	22% patients	STSG
Zeitoun [13]	2002	107[1] (31 Baha)	214 obs.	≤17	8% obs.	11.2% implants	–	STSG
Lloyd [14]	2007	85	4.5 years	<18	46% patients	23.5% patients	42% patients	STSG, FTSG
de Wolf [3]	2008	93	457 obs.	≤16	22.3% obs.	16.3% implants	17% implants	single incision
McDermott [11]	2009	182	15 years	≤16	17% patients	14% implants	–	STSG, pedicled STSG

[1]Includes patients with bone-anchored auricular prosthesis.

Reasons for Soft Tissue Complications

Nature of the Implant

The transcutaneous implant allows constant communication with the external environment. It is also a foreign body. Histologic studies of skin surrounding implants indicate that the number of inflammatory cells is increased even in the absence of clinical signs of inflammation [39, 40]. T-lymphocytes and B-lymphocytes are preferentially accumulated within 1 mm of the interface of implants without clinical evidence of irritation [39]. Inflammation or infection of the implant may occur when there is either a breakdown in this defense mechanism, or the immune system is overwhelmed by the antigenic load. When irritation of the skin becomes clinically evident, there are increased numbers of B-lymphocytes surrounding the implant [40] and often *Staphylococcus aureus* is evident at the site of skin penetration [41]. This inflammatory response does not include a significant increase in T-lymphocytes, which is more suggestive of a response to exogenous factors rather than a chronic allergic response to the implant [39]. A contact allergy to titanium is rare, but has been reported from a pacemaker [42] and was suspected in 1 case of a Baha with chronic inflammation requiring explantation [8].

Increased Thickness of the Scalp

Increased scalp thickness has been linked to increased soft tissue complications. Berenholz et al. [43] found that patients with a BMI greater than 30 had an increased rate of soft tissue complications. In 88 Baha patients, 10 had soft tissue overgrowth of their implant, and 9 of those 10 had a BMI greater than 30 [43]. In a series of 891 patients, Monksfield et al. [44] fitted 81 (9%) patients with a longer abutment (8.5 mm) due to significant soft tissue overgrowth. Of these patients, 98.8% required no further surgical intervention. Although 40 patients had surgical soft tissue reduction prior to placement of the longer abutment, 41 patients were not treated surgically prior to switching to the longer abutment. Men were statistically more likely than women to have soft tissue complications. Berenholz et al. [43] found that men with a BMI >30 were significantly more likely to have complications than women of the same BMI group. Monksfield et al. [44] found that patients who required the longer abutment were predominantly male (64:24 male to female ratio). It is not known why men are more prone to skin overgrowth, but it might be that androgens may increase the tendency toward hypertrophic scarring and that estrogens may exert an anti-inflammatory beneficial role in wound healing [43]. A lower threshold to placing a longer abutment in men with a BMI >30 is being advocated.

Comorbidities
It is likely that medical comorbidities that influence wound healing would result in higher complication rates in patients implanted with a Baha. There are no studies large enough to report any statistical association between soft tissue complications and diabetes, smoking, hypertrophic scarring, or other dermatologic or systemic conditions which might contribute to delayed or retarded wound healing. So contraindications to implantation in these patients are judged on a case by case basis.

Avoiding Soft Tissue Complications

Incision Type: Dermatome versus Single Incision
The benefit of a single incision has already been discussed above with regard to flap necrosis. Some studies have reported no difference in the complication rate comparing the single incision to the grafts and flaps, while others showed a reduction in overall complications. Reduced complications included skin reactions, implant extrusions, abscesses, and number of unscheduled visits [33, 45].

Adequate Soft Tissue Reduction
The subcutaneous tissue must be aggressively removed from above the hair follicles all the way down, with preservation of the periostium. This prevents mobility between the graft/flap and the periostium, which would prevent healing, promote inflammation, and encourage the formation of thick scar tissue. The removal of subcutaneous tissue to as much as 2 cm circumferentially around the implant is necessary. Wider excisions are necessary in the overweight or obese patient.

Hygiene
Regular cleaning is the most effective way to prevent soft tissue reactions. This is best performed daily with soap, water, and a soft brush. Overzealous cleaning on the other hand is a cause for many soft tissue reactions, and patients must be educated, often repeatedly, regarding proper cleaning around the implant.

Conclusion

Osseointegrated bone conduction implants have proven to be safe and effective in the treatment of conductive and mixed hearing losses as well as in single-sided deafness. Successful surgery is predicated upon proper patient selection, appropriate location of the implant, strict handling of the implant, the creation of a thin hair-free immobile flap, and generous wide subcutaneous tissue thinning. Observing experienced surgeons and following the above principles will help newcomers to the field reduce their complication rates and maximize success.

References

1 Wazen JJ, Young DL, Farrugia MC, Chandrasekhar SS, Ghossaini SH, Borik J, Soneru C, Spitzer JB: Successes and complications of the Baha system. Otol Neurotol 2008;29:1115–1119.
2 Albrektsson T, Brånemark PI, Hansson HA, Linström J: Osseointegrated titanium implants: requirements for ensuring a long-lasting, direct bone-to-implant anchorage in man. Acta Orthop Scand 1981;52:155.
3 de Wolf MJF, Hol MKS, Huygen PLM, Mylanus EAM, Cremers CWRJ: Clinical outcome of the simplified surgical technique for BAHA implantation. Otol Neurotol 2008;29:1100–1108.
4 McDermott AM, Sheehan P: Bone-anchored hearing aids in children. Curr Opin Otolaryngol Head Neck Surg 2009; 17:488–493.
5 Proops DW: The Birmingham bone anchored hearing aid programme: surgical methods and complications. J Laryngol Otol 1996;21:7–12.
6 Reyes RA, Tjellström A, Granström G: Evaluation of implant losses and skin reactions around extraoral bone-anchored implants: a 0 to 8 year follow-up. Otolaryngol Head Neck Surg 2000;122:272–276.
7 Tjellström A, Granström G: Long-term follow-up with the bone-anchored hearing aid: a review of the first 100 patients between 1977 and 1985. Ear Nose Throat J 1994;73:112–114.
8 House JW, Kutz JW: Bone-anchored hearing aids: incidence and management of postoperative complications. Otol Neurotol 2007;28:213–217.
9 Tjellström A, Granström G: One-stage procedure to establish osseointegration: a zero to five years follow-up report. J Laryngol Otol 1995;109:593–598.
10 Wazen JL, Caruso M, Tjellström A: Long-term results with the titanium bone-anchored hearing aid: the US experience. Otol Neuotol 1998;19: 737–741.
11 McDermott A, Williams J, Kuo M, Reid A, Proops D: The Birmingham pediatric bone-anchored hearing aid program: a 15-year experience. Otol Neurotol 2009; 30:178–183.
12 Faber HT, de Wolf MJ, de Rooy JWJ, Hol MKS, Cremers CWR, Mylanus EAM: Bone-anchored hearing aid implant location in relation to skin reactions. Arch Otolaryngol Head Neck Surg 2009; 135:742–747.
13 Zeitoun H, Phil M, Ranit D, Thompson S, Proops D: Osseointegrated implants in the management of childhood ear abnormalities: with particular emphasis on complications. J Laryngol Otol 2002; 116:87–91.
14 Lloyd S, Almeyda J, Sirimanna KS, Albert DM, Bailey CM: Updated surgical experience with bone-anchored hearing aids in children. J Laryngol Otol 2007; 121:826–831.
15 Granström G, Bergström K, Odersjö M, Tjellström A: Osseointegrated implants in children: experience from our first 100 patients. Otolaryngol Head Neck Surg 2001;125:85–92.
16 Jacobsson M, Albrektsson T, Tjellström A: Tissue-integrated implants in children. Int J Pediatr Otorhinolaryngol 1992;24:235–243.
17 Davids T, Gordon KA, Clutton D, Papsin BC: Bone-anchored hearing aids in infants and children younger than 5 years. Arch Otolaryngol Head Neck Surg 2007;133:51–55.
18 Badran K, Arya AK, Bunstone D, Mackinnon N: Long-term complications of bone-anchored hearing aids: a 14-year experience. J Laryngol Otol 2009;123: 170–176.
19 Stevenson DS, Proops DW, Wake MJC, et al: Osseointegrated implants in the management of childhood ear abnormalities: the initial Birmingham experience. J Laryngol Otol 1993;107:502–509.
20 Priwin C, Ganström G: The bone-anchored hearing aid in children: a surgical and questionnaire follow-up study. Otolaryngol Head Neck Surg 2005;132: 559–565.
21 Berend N, Kellet B, Kent N, Sly PD: Improved safety with equivalent asthma control in adults with chronics severe asthma on high-dose fluticasone propionate. Respirology 2001;6:237–246.
22 Lipworth BJ: Systemic adverse effects of inhaled corticosteroid therapy: a systemic review and meta-analysis. Arch Intern Med 1999;159:941–955.
23 Wicke C, Halliday B, Allen D, et al: Effects of steroids and retinoids on wound healing. Arch Surg 2000;135: 1265–1270.
24 Krueger JK, Rohrich RJ: Clearing the smoke: the scientific rationale for tobacco abstention with plastic surgery. Plast Reconstr Surg 2001;108: 1063–1077.
25 McCracken M, Lemons JE, Rahemtulla F, Prince CW, Feldman D: Bone response to titanium alloy implants placed in diabetic rats. Int J Oral Maxillofac Implants 2000;15:345–354.
26 Shirazi MA, Marzo SJ, Leonetti JP: Perioperative complications with the bone-anchored hearing aid. Otolaryngol Head Neck Surg 2006;134:236–239.
27 Uppal H, D'Souza A, Proops D: Osseointegration in Paget's disease: the bone-anchored hearing aid in the rehabilitation of Pagetic deafness. J Laryngol Otol 2001;115:903–906.
28 Granström G: Rehabilitation of irradiated cancer patients with tissue-integrated prostheses: adjunctive use of hyperbaric oxygen to improve osseointegration. J Facial Somato Prosthetics 1997;1:1–11.
29 Scholz M, Eufinger H, Anders A, Illerhaus B, Konig M, Schmieder K, Harders A: Intracerebral abscess after abutment change of a bone anchored hearing aid (BAHA). Otol Neurotol 2003;24:896–899.
30 de Wolf MJF, Hol MKS, Mylanus EAM, Cremers CWRJ: Bone-anchored hearing aid surgery in older adults: implant loss and skin reactions. Ann Otolaryngology Rhinol Laryngol 2009;118:525–531.
31 Hobson C, Roper AJ, Andrew R, Rothera MR, Hill P, Green KM: Complications of bone-anchored hearing aid implantation. J Otolaryngol Otol 2010;124: 132–136.
32 Tjellström A, Granstrom G: How we do it: frequency of skin necrosis after BAHA surgery. Clin Otolaryngol 2006;31: 216–232.
33 Mudry A: Bone-anchored hearing aids (BAHA): skin healing process for skin flap technique versus linear incision technique in the first three months after the implantation. Rev Larynogol Otol Rhinol 2009;130:281–284.

34 Holgers KM, Tjellström A, Bjursten LM, Erlandsson BE: Soft tissue reactions around percutaneous implants: a clinical study of soft tissue conditions around skin-penetrating titanium implants for bone-anchored hearing aids. Am J Otol 1988;9:56–59.
35 Falcone MT, Kaylie DM, Labadie RF, Haynes DS: Bone-anchored hearing aid abutment skin overgrowth reduction with clobetasol. Otolaryngol Head Neck Surg 2008;139:829–832.
36 Mylanus EA, Johansson CB, Cremers CW: Craniofacial titanium implants and chronic pain: histologic findings. Otol Neurotol 2002;23:920–925.
37 Doshi J, McDermott AL, Proops D: The use of a bone-anchored hearing aid (Baha) in children with severe behavioural problems – The Birmingham Baha programme experience. Int J Ped Otorhinolaryngol 2010;74:608–610.
38 Sheehan PZ, Hols PS: UK and Ireland experience of bone-anchored hearing aids (BAHA) in individuals with Down's syndrome. Int J Pediat Otorhinolaryngol 2006;70:981–986.
39 Holgers KM: Characteristics of the inflammatory process around skin-penetrating titanium implants for aural rehabilitation. Audiology 2000;39: 253–259.
40 Holgers KM, Thomsen P, Tjellström A, Bjursten LM: Immunohistochemical study of the soft tissue around long-term skin-penetrating titanium implants. Biomaterials 1995;16:611–616.
41 Holgers KM, Thomsen P, Tjellström A, Ericson LE: Electron microscopical observations on the soft tissue in clinical long-term percutaneous titanium implants. Biomaterials 1995;16:83–90.
42 Yamauchi R, Morita A, Tsuji T: Pacemaker dermatitis from titanium. Contact Dermatitis 2000;42:52–53.
43 Berenholz LP, Burkey JM, Lippy WH: High body mass index as a risk factor for skin overgrowth with the bone-anchored hearing aid. Otol Neurotol 2010;31: 430–432.
44 Monksfield P, Ho EC, Reid A, Proops D: Experience with the longer (8.5 mm) abutment for bone-anchored hearing aid. Otol Neurotol 2009;30:274–276.
45 Van de Berg R, Stokroos RJ, Hof JR, Chenault MN: Bone-anchored hearing aid: a comparison of surgical techniques. Otol Neurotol 2009;31:129–135.

Jack J. Wazen, MD
Silverstein Institute, Ear Research Foundation
1901 Floyd Street
Sarasota, FL 34239 (USA)
Tel. +1 941 366 9222, E-Mail otonro@gmail.com

Kompis M, Caversaccio M-D (eds): Implantable Bone Conduction Hearing Aids.
Adv Otorhinolaryngol. Basel, Karger, 2011, vol 71, pp 73–83

Audiological Results with Baha® in Conductive and Mixed Hearing Loss

Flurin Pfiffner · Marco-Domenico Caversaccio · Martin Kompis

Department of ENT, Head and Neck Surgery, Inselspital, University of Bern, Bern, Switzerland

Abstract

The level of improvement in the audiological results of Baha® users mainly depends on the patient's preoperative hearing thresholds and the type of Baha sound processor used. This investigation shows correlations between the preoperative hearing threshold and postoperative aided thresholds and audiological results in speech understanding in quiet of 84 Baha users with unilateral conductive hearing loss, bilateral conductive hearing loss and bilateral mixed hearing loss. Secondly, speech understanding in noise of 26 Baha users with different Baha sound processors (Compact, Divino, and BP100) is investigated. Linear regression between aided sound field thresholds and bone conduction (BC) thresholds of the better ear shows highest correlation coefficients and the steepest slope. Differences between better BC thresholds and aided sound field thresholds are smallest for mid-frequencies (1 and 2 kHz) and become larger at 0.5 and 4 kHz. For Baha users, the gain in speech recognition in quiet can be expected to lie in the order of magnitude of the gain in their hearing threshold. Compared to its predecessor sound processors Baha® Compact and Baha® Divino, Baha® BP100 improves speech understanding in noise significantly by +0.9 to +4.6 dB signal-to-noise ratio, depending on the setting and the use of directional microphone. For Baha users with unilateral and bilateral conductive hearing loss and bilateral mixed hearing loss, audiological results in aided sound field thresholds can be estimated with the better BC hearing threshold. The benefit in speech understanding in quiet can be expected to be similar to the gain in their sound field hearing threshold. The most recent technology of Baha sound processor improves speech understanding in noise by an order of magnitude that is well perceived by users and which can be very useful in everyday life.

The Baha® system [1] that enables sound transmission by direct bone conduction (BC) [2] from the retroauricular implant to the inner ear has been in clinical use since 1977 [3]. A large number of studies on outcomes with the Baha system in cases of conductive and mixed hearing loss have been published [4–13] and show significant benefits to sound field hearing thresholds, in speech understanding and subjective user ratings.

A prediction of audiological results before a patient undergoes surgery is very desirable for patients and useful to determine potential Baha candidates. The most common method to estimate the benefit of a Baha system is to attach the Baha sound processor to a soft band or headband that is provided by the manufacturer. After fitting of the

Baha sound processor, the Baha candidates can use the system in an everyday situation and can evaluate the subjective benefits. However, if the Baha sound processor is attached to a test band and not directly to the implant, the transmission of sound to the inner ear is damped by soft tissue by approximately 10–20 dB [2] resulting in poorer audiological outcomes [14].

Another method to predict the audiological results with Baha is to analyze the correlation between the preoperative pure tone audiogram and the postoperative outcomes of Baha users, i.e. sound field hearing thresholds as well as speech reception thresholds (SRTs). This prediction of Baha outcomes is influenced by different factors, e.g. position of Baha implant [15], hearing loss indication of Baha users (e.g. conductive or mixed hearing loss), type of Baha sound processor (e.g. Baha® Compact, the Baha® Divino, Baha® Intenso or Baha® BP100 [16, 17] and settings of the Baha sound processor controls (e.g. the omnidirectional versus the directional microphone mode [8]). Data from Pfiffner et al. [13] show correlations between preoperative pure tone hearing thresholds and postoperative aided sound field hearing threshold as a function of different hearing loss indications, i.e. Baha users with single-sided deafness, unilateral and bilateral conductive hearing loss.

In this chapter, we present an overview of audiological results with Baha in conductive and mixed hearing loss. It first investigates correlations between audiological results with the Baha system and preoperative pure tone thresholds for these different patient indications, i.e. correlations between preoperative pure tone hearing thresholds and postoperative aided sound field hearing threshold are analyzed, and then correlations between audiological results in speech understanding benefit and functional gain are investigated. Finally, it investigates audiological results of speech understanding in noise for Baha users as a function of different Baha processors.

Materials and Methods

Subjects
Adult subjects were selected from patients who had been implanted and fitted with the Baha system at the University ENT Department of the Inselspital in Bern. Selection criteria for inclusion in this retrospective study were that subjects had to be German speaking and use a Baha system unilaterally.

Audiological Measurements
Preoperative pure tone audiograms were measured for all Baha users, including measurement of air conduction (AC) and BC hearing thresholds in both ears. If necessary, insert phones and narrow band noise masking was used to identify hearing thresholds for each ear unambiguously.

The audiological results of the Baha system were evaluated 3 months after first fitting of the sound processor. Benefits of sound field hearing thresholds were measured at 0.5, 1, 2 and 4 kHz using narrow band noise. To determine speech understanding in quiet, two-digit German numbers and monosyllabic words from the Swiss version of the German Freiburg Test were evaluated in sound field for aided and unaided conditions [18]. According to the standard test procedure, the 50% SRT was measured for two-digit numbers and recognition scores at 50, 65 and 80 dB were determined for monosyllabic words. Speech understanding in noise was measured with either the Basler [19] or with the Oldenburger Sentence Test [20]. The standard adaptive test procedure was applied to determine the signal-to-noise ratio (SNR), where 50% of speech understanding in noise was obtained. Speech understanding in noise was measured in two different spatial settings: with both the target and the noise signal coming from the front (S0N0), or with the target sentences arriving from the front but the noise coming from the rear of the subject (S0N180).

Analysis of Audiological Results
The first audiological results included outcomes of 84 out of 322 Baha users that were divided into three groups according to their preoperative indication (table 1), i.e. unilateral conductive hearing loss, bilateral conductive hearing loss and bilateral mixed hearing loss.

Group A (unilateral conductive hearing loss) comprised 24 Baha users:

- with normal or almost normal hearing threshold in the Baha contralateral ear, i.e. if the AC hearing threshold averaged over the frequencies of 0.5, 1, 2, and 4 kHz, was better than 40 dB and any air-bone gap (ABG), if present, was smaller than 20 dB;
- with a conductive hearing loss in the Baha ear side, i.e. if the averaged AC hearing threshold was 40 dB or more and the averaged ABG was 20 dB or more.

Table 1. Included groups of Baha users according to their preoperative hearing indication

	Hearing indication at Baha ear	Hearing indication at contralateral ear	Subjects (female/male)	Age, years
Group A, unilateral conductive hearing loss	conductive hearing loss[1]	normal hearing[2]	24 (12/12)	50.6 (21–74)
Group B, bilateral conductive hearing loss	conductive hearing loss[1]	conductive hearing loss[1]	38 (16/22)	42.9 (19–85)
Group C, bilateral mixed hearing loss	mixed hearing loss[3]	mixed hearing loss[3]	22 (15/7)	68 (29–87)

Values for age are expressed as mean (range).
[1]Defined as PTA_{BC} <30 dB HL and PTA_{AC} >40 dB HL or PTA_{AC} <40 dB HL and ABG >20.
[2]Defined as PTA_{AC} <40 dB HL and ABG <20 dB.
[3]Defined as better PTA_{AC} >35 dB HL and ABG ≥20 and better PTA_{BC} >20 dB HL.

Table 2. Synopsis of the Baha user groups included in speech understanding in noise investigation

Comparison of sound processor Baha Divino (omnidirectional) with	Subjects (female/male)	Age, years (mean (range))	Speech test
Baha Compact	7 (4/3)	49 (19–66)	Basler Sentence Test
Baha Divino (directional)	26 (14/12)	50 (19–72)	Basler or Oldenburger Sentence Test
Baha BP100 (omnidirectional)	19 (10/9)	51 (22–72)	Oldenburger Sentence Test
Baha BP100 (directional)	19 (10/9)	51 (22–72)	Oldenburger Sentence Test

Values for age are expressed as mean (range).

Group B (bilateral conductive hearing loss) comprised 38 Baha users with a bilateral conductive hearing loss as defined above.

Group C (bilateral mixed hearing loss) comprised 22 subjects with a bilateral mixed hearing loss, i.e. if the average over the frequencies of 0.5, 1, 2, and 4 kHz BC hearing threshold was poorer than 20 dB, the average AC hearing threshold was poorer than 35 dB HL and the average ABG was larger than 20 dB.

The second part of audiological results present speech understanding in noise scores of 26 Baha users. These audiological results of Baha users with bilateral conductive or bilateral hearing loss are presented as a function of the three sound processors Baha Compact, Baha Divino and Baha BP100 (table 2). Data include 7 Baha users from a comparative study between Baha Compact and Baha Divino [8] and 19 Baha users from an ongoing prospective comparative study of Baha BP100 and Baha Divino. All SNR are standardized to the SNR results with the Baha Divino in the omnidirectional microphone mode (benefit in SNR = 0) in order to have comparative results.

Data were analyzed using the Prism 5.03/Instat 3.05 software package (GraphPad Inc., San Diego, Calif., USA).

Baha Sound Processors and Settings
Included subjects used their everyday settings for all measurements of audiological outcomes and did not change the sound processor settings [21, 22]. It has previously been shown that there is no significant difference between the two sound processors Baha Compact and Baha Divino

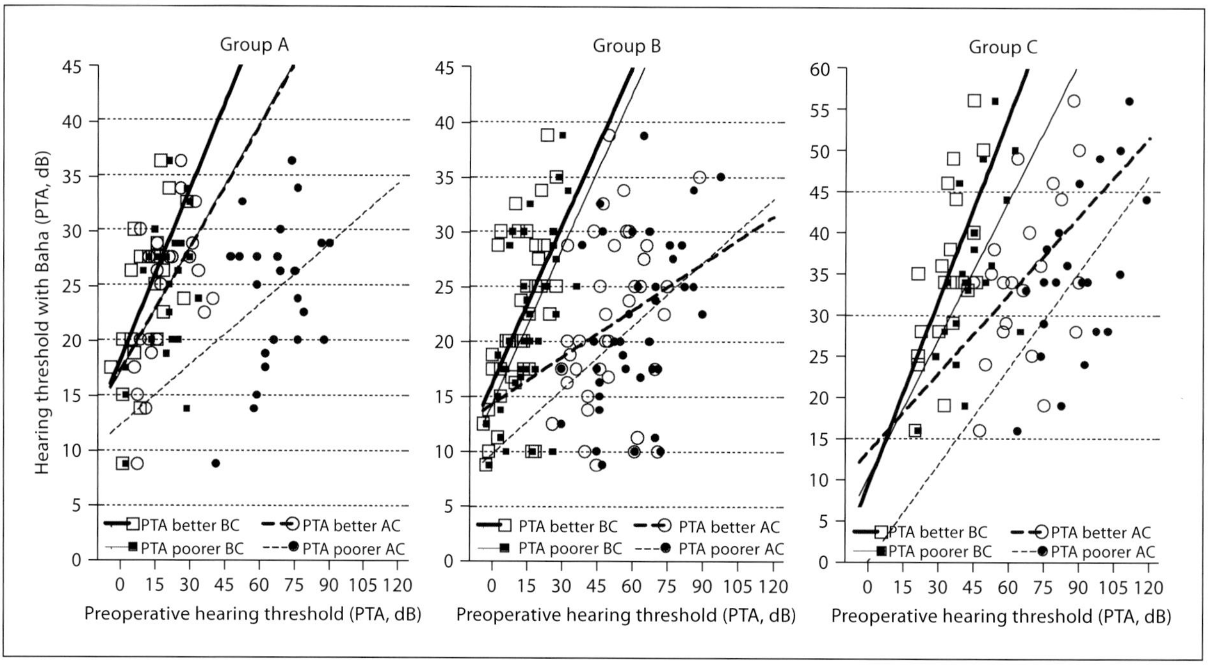

Fig. 1. Individual audiological outcomes in aided sound field (y-axis) as a function of preoperative hearing thresholds (x-axis). Linear regressions are shown for each preoperative hearing threshold (better and poorer AC and BC thresholds) of the three study groups. PTA was measured over the frequencies of 0.5, 1, 2, and 4 kHz.

when comparing aided sound field thresholds and speech reception in quiet [8]. All subjects in groups A and B were fitted with either a Baha Compact sound processor or a Baha Divino sound processor. Five subjects of group C used a Baha Intenso sound processor as proposed by the manufacturer in cases of substantial mixed hearing loss [21]. All subjects included in the study had a minimum 3 months' experience with Baha.

Subjects that participated in the audiological evaluation of speech understanding in noise used their sound processor Baha Compact and then for at least 3 months the Baha Divino, or the Baha Divino and then for at least 3 months the Baha BP100.

Results

The correlations between the audiological results of aided sound field hearing threshold (y-axis) and preoperative bone and AC hearing thresholds of both ears (x-axis) are presented in figure 1. Individual data of all subjects are shown in a different figure according to their hearing loss indication (group A, B and C). The correlation coefficients and the level of statistical significance are summarized in table 3.

For group A (unilateral conductive hearing loss group) [13], the best correlation coefficient is obtained between the PTA (pure tone average) of the ears with the better BC and the aided hearing threshold. This correlation curve shows the steepest slope. In contrast, there is no significant correlation between the poorer AC and the aided sound field threshold. The correlation between the poorer BC and the better AC is lower, but still statistically significant.

For group B (bilateral conductive hearing loss) [13], the slopes of poorer and better BC differ

Table 3. Correlation coefficients (r^2) and level of statistical significance (*$p < 0.05$, **$p < 0.01$, ***$p < 0.001$) for linear regression between audiological results with Baha in sound field and preoperative hearing thresholds of AC and BC of better and poorer ear

Linear regression between aided sound field threshold and	Group A	Group B	Group C
Better BC	$r^2 = 0.419$*** $p = 0.0006$	$r^2 = 0.319$*** $p = 0.0002$	$r^2 = 0.425$** $p = 0.0014$
Poorer BC	$r^2 = 0.248$* $p = 0.0133$	$r^2 = 0.376$*** $p < 0.0001$	$r^2 = 0.357$** $p = 0.0042$
Better AC	$r^2 = 0.306$** $p = 0.0051$	$r^2 = 0.073$ $p = 0.1003$	$r^2 = 0.207$* $p = 0.0384$
Poorer AC	$r^2 = 0.117$ $p = 0.102$	$r^2 = 0.170$* $p = 0.0102$	$r^2 = 0.330$** $p = 0.0064$

statistically significantly from 0 ($p < 0.0002$) and correlate relatively highly with the aided threshold. Both AC thresholds correlate less with aided PTAs.

For group C (bilateral mixed hearing loss group), the best correlation exists between the better BC and the aided sound field threshold. Both AC thresholds correlate less with aided PTAs.

In summary, for groups A–C, the correlation curve between the audiological results in aided sound field threshold and the better BC thresholds shows the steepest slope. The aided sound field threshold with Baha correlates best with the better BC thresholds found in pure tone audiometry for groups A and C. Correlations with the BC thresholds of both ears are similar for group B.

The audiological outcomes in aided sound field thresholds (y-axis) are presented as a function of frequency (x-axis) in figure 2. The better BC hearing thresholds are shown as reference values in the same figure. Median value differences are small at 1 and 2 kHz (–7.5 to 10 dB) and increase at 500 Hz (10–17.5 dB) and at 4 kHz (5–15 dB). Median aided sound field thresholds are lower than the BC thresholds at all frequencies for groups A and B [13]. Group C shows better aided hearing thresholds for frequencies at 1 and 2 kHz compared to better BC hearing thresholds.

Figure 3 presents the individual audiological results of SRT benefits of 50% German two-digit number for all included subjects. SRT (y-axis) is correlated with the functional gain, i.e. the difference between aided and unaided hearing threshold in sound field (x-axis). All three study groups were investigated separately. These correlations are statistically highly significant ($p < 0.0001$ for groups A and B, $p = 0.0007$ for group C). All three study groups have approximately the same slopes (range 0.81–1.06).

In summary, for Baha users in groups A–C, the Baha system enables a gain of approximately 0.8–1.1 dB in terms of SRT per dB gain in the PTA sound field threshold.

The averaged best fit curves of aided and unaided speech intelligibility for monosyllabic words are presented in figure 4. The difference between aided and unaided conditions are for the study groups A (24.0 dB) [13], B (26.2 dB) [13], and C (24.2 dB). Presented curves are best fits (least squared error) to the Boltzman sigmoidal function $y = 100\%/(1 + \exp[(a - x)/b])$, where y (%) is the proportion of correctly understood monosyllabic words and

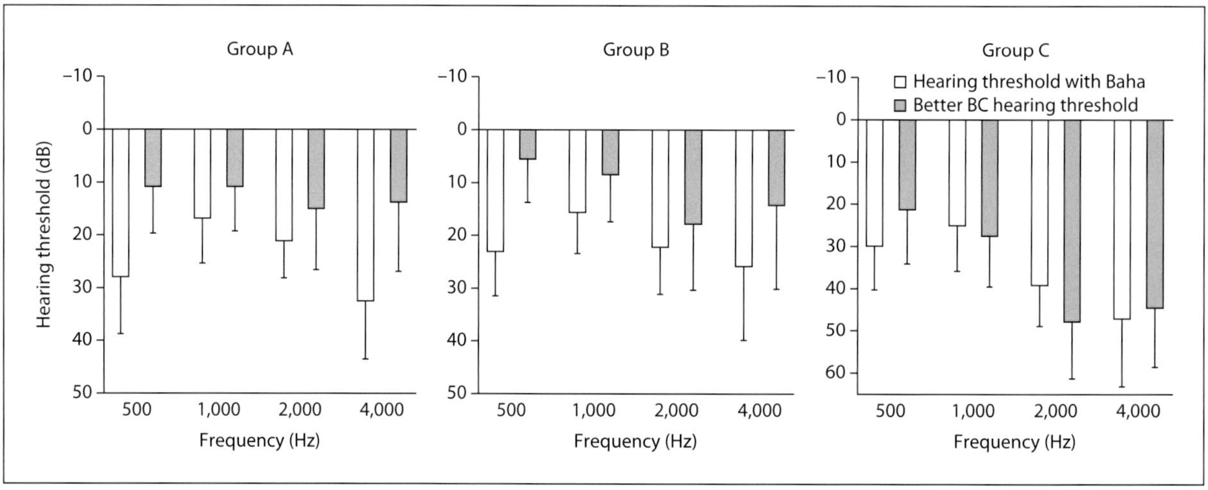

Fig. 2. Hearing threshold relative to 0 dB of aided sound field and better BC over the frequencies of 0.5, 1, 2, and 4 kHz of the three study groups. Bar plots with standard deviation.

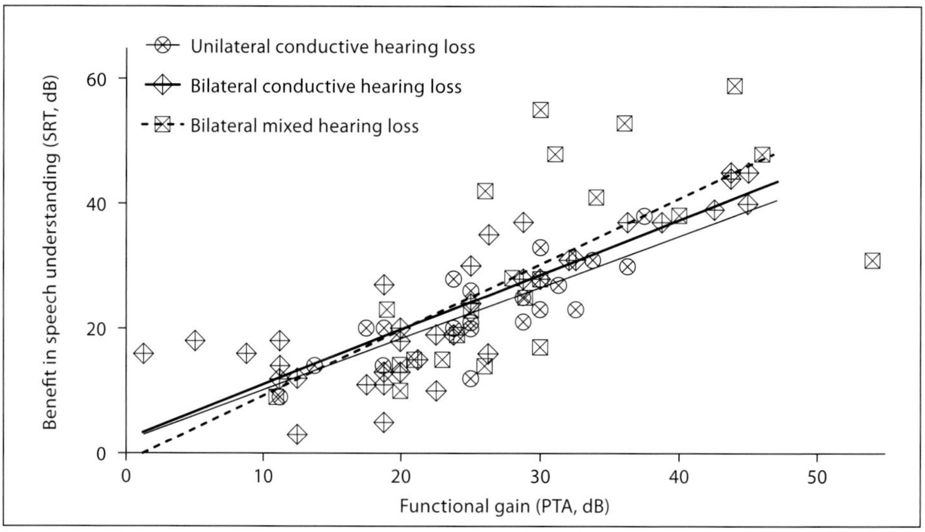

Fig. 3. Individual audiological outcomes in SRT benefit (y-axis) as a function of the gain in sound field with Baha (x-axis). Linear regressions are shown for the three study groups. PTA was measured over the frequencies of 0.5, 1, 2, and 4 kHz.

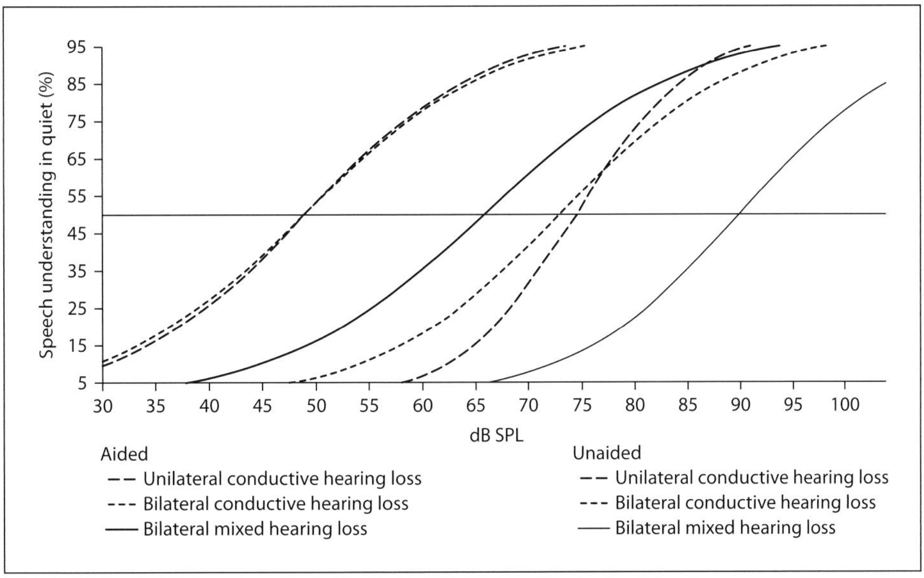

Fig. 4. Audiological outcomes of speech understanding in quiet (y-axis) as a function of the presentation level in dB SPL (x-axis) for the three study groups in aided and unaided situations. The curves are best fits (least squared error) to a Boltzman sigmoidal function.

x (dB SPL) is the presentation level. Parameter a (dB SPL) corresponds to the presentation level for 50% word understanding, and parameter b (%/dB SPL) is the slope of the curve at point a.

Figure 5 shows the speech understanding in noise benefit in dB SNR as a function of the Baha sound processor used (Compact, Divino and BP100). All audiological results are presented relative to the speech performance with the Baha Divino in the omnidirectional microphone mode, i.e. speech performance with the Baha Divino in the omnidirectional mode is standardized to 0 dB SNR benefit.

The Baha Compact sound processor shows the poorest speech understanding in noise compared to the other sound processors in both situations, i.e. noise presented from the rear (–1.2 dB SNR compared to Baha Divino in the omnidirectional mode, fig. 5) and from the front (–0.9 dB SNR compared to Baha Divino in the omnidirectional mode, fig. 5) [8].

Audiological results with the Baha Divino sound processor in the directional microphone mode show significant improvement in speech understanding in noise (+1.9 dB SNR, $p < 0.001$, Wilcoxon matched-pairs signed-rank test) in S0N180 compared to the Baha Divino in the omnidirectional mode.

As can be expected, no significant difference between Baha Divino in the omnidirectional and directional microphone modes is measured in a situation where noise and speech signal are presented from the front (–0.1 dB SNR, Wilcoxon matched-pairs signed-rank test).

The Baha BP100 sound processor shows better speech understanding in noise scores in both conditions (S0N180 and S0N0) and for both microphone modes compared to the Baha Divino. For the Baha BP100, there is a statistically significant benefit in the omnidirectional mode (+2.3 dB SNR, $p < 0.001$, Wilcoxon matched-pairs signed-rank test) and directional microphone (+4.6 dB

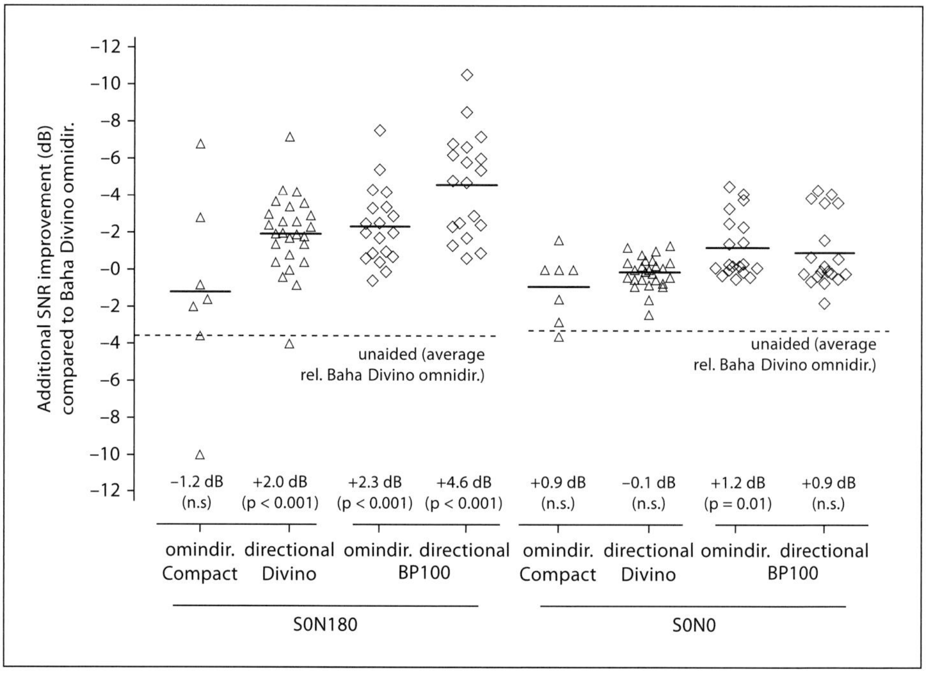

Fig. 5. Benefits of speech understanding in noise (ΔdB SNR for 50% speech understanding unaided compared to aided) with different speech processors shown as improvement compared to the Baha Divino in the omnidirectional microphone mode (speech understanding performance with the Baha Divino in the omnidirectional mode is standardized to 0 dB SNR benefit). Left: target sentences arriving from the front and the noise coming from the rear (S0N180). Right: target and the noise signal coming from the front (S0N0).

SNR, $p < 0.001$, Wilcoxon matched-pairs signed-rank test) compared to the Baha Divino in the omnidirectional mode, if the noise signal arrives from the rear (S0N180). In condition S0N0, the benefit is 1.2 dB ($p = 0.01$, Wilcoxon matched-pairs signed-rank test) and 0.9 dB (n.s., Wilcoxon matched-pairs signed-rank test), respectively, compared to the Baha Divino in the omnidirectional mode.

Discussion

Audiological Results: Sound Field Hearing Thresholds

As could be expected, audiological results with the Baha system correlated with preoperative hearing thresholds. Understanding this correlation is extremely useful prior to surgery when estimating a predicted improvement in audiological results. The best correlation and the highest slope can be found between the better BC threshold and the aided sound field threshold (table 3; fig. 1). Only in the case of group B (bilateral conductive hearing loss) are similar correlations and slopes for the BC threshold of either the better or the poorer ear determined. For each group, the aided sound field hearing thresholds can be estimated as a function of the better BC threshold as follows:

For unilateral conductive hearing loss (group A):

$$\text{Aided sound field hearing thresholds} \approx 18.1\ \text{dB} + 0.52 \cdot \text{PTA BC,better ear} \qquad (1)$$

For bilateral conductive hearing loss (group B):

Aided sound field hearing thresholds ≈
16.1 dB + 0.48 · PTA BC, better ear (2)

For bilateral mixed hearing loss (group C):

Aided sound field hearing thresholds ≈
9.5 dB + 0.33 · PTA BC, better ear (3)

With these formulae, the aided PTA is predicted correctly within ±10 dB for approximately 83% of the subjects and for 58% even within ±5 dB. In order to have a simple formula for everyday use, the coefficient can be rounded:

If BC threshold better ear <25 dB:

Aided sound field hearing thresholds ≈
17 dB + 1/2 · PTA BC, better ear (4)

If BC threshold better ear >25 dB:

Aided sound field hearing thresholds ≈
10 dB + 1/3 · PTA BC, better ear (5)

The frequency dependency between aided and unaided better BC thresholds is shown in figure 2. Aided sound field thresholds are best for mid-frequencies (1 and 2 kHz) compared to better BC thresholds. These results are comparable with earlier studies [2, 8, 13, 15] and can be explained by the physical characteristics of the sound processor with a maximal output force around 1 kHz. In group C where Baha users have the poorest preoperative BC, the aided thresholds for mid-frequencies are higher than the BC thresholds, i.e. the delivered acoustic energy of the Baha system can partially compensate for the sensorineural hearing loss component. Middle frequencies are of great importance for speech understanding [23].

Audiological Results: Speech Understanding in Quiet

Improvement in sound field thresholds correlates with improvements in SRTs in quiet of two-digit numbers (fig. 3) and monosyllabic words (fig. 4).

For each group, speech understanding of two-digit numbers can be estimated as a function of the gain in sound field, i.e. for everyday use a simple formula with rounded coefficient is:

If BC threshold better ear <25 dB:

Correct two- digit numbers (%) ≈
2 + 0.8 (%/dB) · gain in sound field (dB) (6)

If BC threshold better ear >25 dB:

Correct two- digit numbers (%) ≈
1(%/dB) · gain in sound field (dB) (7)

Using formula 6, results for speech understanding of all subjects (group A and B) are better or in the range of –5%. Formula 7 predicts better or results in the range of –5% for 77% of subjects in group C.

Audiological results for 50% monosyllabic word understanding in aided and unaided conditions (fig. 4) show an average difference of 24.0 dB (group A), 26.2 dB (group B), and 24.2 dB (group C), and are close to the respective mean improvements in sound field thresholds of 25.9, 24.1 and 29.4 dB. Audiological results of both speech understanding tests show that the gain in sound field is a reasonable estimation parameter for sound reception in quiet.

Audiological Results: Speech Understanding in Noise

It is expected that speech understanding in noise is increased when directional microphones are used in situations with noise from the rear (S0N180). Our findings (+2.0 dB SNR Baha Divino and +4.6 dB SNR Baha BP100; fig. 5) are in line with other studies comparing two-microphone noise reduction systems in conventional hearing aids with improvement from +1.5 to +8.5 dB SNR [24–27].

Further, the audiological results of our investigations show that speech understanding in noise depends on the type of sound processor. Poorest speech understanding in noise is measured with the Baha Compact in both situations (S0N180: –1.2 dB SNR and S0N0: –0.9 dB SNR) compared to the Baha Divino in the omnidirectional microphone mode. The Baha BP100 sound processor provides better speech understanding in noise in situations when noise presented from the rear (S0N180: +2.3 to +4.6 dB SNR) and from the front (S0N0: +0.9 to +1.2 dB SNR) compared to the Baha Divino in the omnidirectional microphone mode. Several technical improvements might explain the difference between the Baha Divino and BP100: measurement of the direct BC with the Baha BP100 fitting software [22], the position compensation, adjustment of the individual gain in 10 frequency bands, and the wide dynamic range compression in the BP100 versus a much simpler AGC-O in the Baha Divino.

Conclusions

The preoperative BC threshold is useful to estimate audiological results in aided sound field thresholds of Baha users with unilateral and bilateral conductive hearing loss and bilateral mixed hearing loss. The benefit in speech understanding in quiet can be expected to be similar to the gain in their sound field hearing threshold. The most recent technology of Baha sound processor increases speech understanding in noise by an order of magnitude that is well perceived by users and which can be very useful in everyday life.

Acknowledgements

This work was supported by the department of clinical research of the University of Bern, the Swiss Commission of Technology and Innovation grant No. 8075.1. We would like to thank Ms. Lindsay Bruce for proofreading the manuscript.

References

1 Hakansson B, Tjellstrom A, Rosenhall U, Carlsson P: The bone-anchored hearing aid. Principal design and a psychoacoustical evaluation. Acta Otolaryngol 1985; 100:229–239.

2 Hakansson B, Tjellstrom A, Rosenhall U: Hearing thresholds with direct bone conduction versus conventional bone conduction. Scand Audiol 1984;13:3–13.

3 Tjellstrom A, Rosenhall U, Lindstrom J, Hallen O, Albrektsson T, Branemark PI: Five-year experience with skin-penetrating bone-anchored implants in the temporal bone. Acta Otolaryngol 1983;95:568–575.

4 Hakansson B, Liden G, Tjellstrom A: Ten years of experience with the Swedish bone-anchored hearing system. Ann Otol Rhinol Laryngol Suppl 1990;151: 1–16.

5 Tjellstrom A, Hakansson B: The bone-anchored hearing aid. Design principles, indications, and long-term clinical results. Otolaryngol Clin North Am 1995;28:53–72.

6 Negri S, Bernath O, Hausler R: Bone conduction implants: Xomed Audiant bone conductor vs. BAHA. Ear Nose Throat J 1997;76:394–396.

7 Lustig LR, Arts HA, Brackmann DE: Hearing rehabilitation using the BAHA bone-anchored hearing aid: results in 40 patients. Otol Neurotol 2001;22: 328–334.

8 Kompis M, Krebs M, Hausler R: Speech understanding in quiet and in noise with the bone-anchored hearing aids Baha Compact and Baha Divino. Acta Otolaryngol 2007;127:829–835.

9 Kunst SJ, Leijendeckers JM, Mylanus EA, Hol MK, Snik AF, Cremers CW: Bone-anchored hearing aid system application for unilateral congenital conductive hearing impairment: audiometric results. Otol Neurotol 2008;29:2–7.

10 Priwin C, Jonsson R, Hultcrantz M, Granstrom G: BAHA in children and adolescents with unilateral or bilateral conductive hearing loss: a study of outcome. Int J Pediatr Otorhinolaryngol 2007;71:135–145.

11 Snik AF, Bosman AJ, Mylanus EA, Cremers CW: Candidacy for the bone-anchored hearing aid. Audiol Neurootol 2004;9:190–196.

12 Wazen JJ, Caruso M, Tjellstrom A: Long-term results with the titanium bone-anchored hearing aid: the U.S. experience. Am J Otol 1998;19:737–741.

13 Pfiffner F, Kompis M, Stieger C: Bone-anchored hearing aids: correlation between pure-tone thresholds and outcome in three user groups. Otol Neurotol 2009;30:884–890.

14 Grunder I, Seidl RO, Ernst A, Todt I: Relative value of BAHA testing for the postoperative audiological outcome (in German). HNO 2008;56:1020–1024.

15 Stenfelt S, Hakansson B, Tjellstrom A: Vibration characteristics of bone conducted sound in vitro. J Acoust Soc Am 2000;107:422–431.

16 Entific Medical Systems: Good Things Come in Small Packages! Bone Anchored Applications. Entific Medical Systems, Gothenburg, 2000, vol 2, pp 8–9.

17 Cochlear Bone Anchored Solutions AB: Cochlear™ Baha® Product Catalogue. Mölnlycke, Cochlear Bone Anchored Solutions AB, 2010.

18 Kompis M, Krebs M, Hausler R: Verification of normative values for the Swiss version of the Freiburg speech intelligibility test. HNO 2006;54:445–450.

19 Niklès JM, Tschopp K: Audiologische Grundlagen des Basler Satztests. Audiol Akust 1996;2:70–75.

20 Kollmeier B: Handbuch und Hintergrundwissen: Oldenburger Satztest. Oldenburg, Universität Oldenburg, 2000, pp 1–16.

21 Cochlear Bone Anchored Solutions AB: Baha® Fitting Guide. Mölnlycke, Cochlear Bone Anchored Solutions AB, 2008.

22 Cochlear Bone Anchored Solutions AB: Cochlear™ Baha® Fitting Software 1.0 Guide. Mölnlycke, Cochlear Bone Anchored Solutions AB, 2009.

23 ANSI S3.5–1997: American National Standards Methods for Calculation of the Speech Intelligibility Index. New York, American National Standards Institute, 1997.

24 Lurquin P, Rafhay S: Intelligibility in noise using multi-microphone hearing aids. Acta Otorhinolaryngol 1996;50:103–109.

25 Maj JB, Wouters J, Moonen M: Noise reduction results of an adaptive filtering technique for dual-microphone behind-the-ear hearing aids. Ear Hear 2004;25: 215–229.

26 Valente M, Schuchman G, Potts LG, Beck LB: Performance of dual-microphone in-the-ear hearing aids. J Am Acad Audiol 2000;11:181–189.

27 Valente M, Fabry DA, Potts LG: Recognition of speech in noise with hearing aids using dual microphones. J Am Acad Audiol 1995;6:440–449.

Flurin Pfiffner, PhD
Department of ENT, Head and Neck Surgery, Inselspital, University of Bern
CH – 3010 Bern (Switzerland)
Tel. +41 31 632 33 00, Fax +41 31 632 31 93, E- Mail flurin.pfiffner@dkf.unibe.ch

Kompis M, Caversaccio M-D (eds): Implantable Bone Conduction Hearing Aids.
Adv Otorhinolaryngol. Basel, Karger, 2011, vol 71, pp 84–91

Conductive Hearing Loss and Bone Conduction Devices: Restored Binaural Hearing?

Martijn J.H. Agterberg[a,b] · Myrthe K.S. Hol[a] · Cor W.R.J. Cremers[a] · Emmanuel A.M. Mylanus[a] · A. John van Opstal[b] · Ad F.M. Snik[a]

[a]Department of Otorhinolaryngology, Donders Institute for Brain, Cognition and Behaviour, Radboud University Medical Centre Nijmegen, [b]Department of Biophysics, Donders Institute for Brain, Cognition and Behaviour, Radboud University Nijmegen, Nijmegen, The Netherlands

Abstract

An important aspect of binaural hearing is the proper detection of interaural sound level differences and interaural timing differences. Assessments of binaural hearing were made in patients with acquired unilateral conductive hearing loss (UCHL, n = 11) or congenital UCHL (n = 10) after unilateral application of a bone conduction device (BCD), and in patients with bilateral conductive or mixed hearing loss after bilateral BCD application. Benefit (bilateral versus unilateral listening) was assessed by measuring directional hearing, compensation of the acoustic head shadow, binaural summation and binaural squelch. Measurements were performed after an acclimatization time of at least 10 weeks. Unilateral BCD application was beneficial, but there was less benefit in the patients with congenital UCHL as compared to patients with acquired UCHL. In adults with bilateral hearing loss, bilateral BCD application was clearly beneficial as compared to unilateral BCD application. Binaural summation was present, but binaural squelch could not be proven. To explain the poor results in the patients with congenital UCHL, two factors seemed to be important. First, a critical period in the development of binaural hearing might affect the binaural hearing abilities. Second, crossover stimulation, referring to additional stimulation of the cochlea contralateral to the BCD side, might deteriorate binaural hearing in patients with UCHL.

In the early 1980s, Hausler et al. [1] and several other research groups studied binaural hearing in patients with conductive hearing loss. They found that sound localization was poor. To improve the hearing of such patients, air conduction hearing aids are an option. However, air conduction devices might cause problems in conductive and mixed hearing loss [2]. Therefore, bone conduction devices (BCDs) might be a better choice. In patients with conductive or mixed hearing loss caused by bony atresia of the external ear canal, or in patients with chronic inflammation, they are the sole established option [3].

An important factor affecting binaural hearing with a BCD is cross-stimulation. This is the additional stimulation, through bone conduction, of the cochlea contralateral of the BCD side. This so called cross-hearing is possible because of the limited transcranial attenuation of sound

Table 1. Group characteristics

Group	Patients	Age, years	PTA dB HL	A-B gap	PTA dB HL	A-B gap
Acquired UCHL	11	46 (10)	13 (5)	–	63 (12)	50 (12)
Congenital UCHL	10	27 (15)	9 (5)	–	65 (10)	50 (9)
Bilateral HL	19	46 (16)	58 (15)	33 (14)	63 (12)	36 (10)

PTA = Mean hearing loss (at 0.5, 1, 2, 4 kHz); A-B gap = mean air-bone gap (at 0.5, 1, 2, 4 kHz). Values for age, PTA and A-B gap are expressed as mean (SD).

vibrations in the skull. It has been established that this transcranial attenuation is in the order of 5–15 dB [4, 5]. Cross-hearing might particularly affect directional hearing since directional hearing in the horizontal (azimuth) plane relies on interaural time differences and interaural level differences.

Studies on subjects with normal hearing, however, showed good directional hearing results when stimuli were presented via bone conductor transducers [6]. MacDonald et al. [7] concluded that in adults with normal hearing, bilateral BCDs effectively displayed spatial information. This suggests that despite the limitations in cochlear isolation with bone conduction stimulation, directional hearing is possible. Thus, fitting of BCDs might be an effective option to restore binaural hearing in patients with unilateral and with bilateral conductive hearing loss. The well-documented advantages of binaural hearing are: (a) Improvement in hearing sensitivity and speech recognition owing to bilateral summation. Inputs received by the two cochleae are added together. Perceived improvement in loudness will be 3–6 dB, which results in better speech recognition. (b) Improvement in speech recognition in noisy situations with spatially separated speech and noise sources. (c) Improved directional hearing.

Initial measurements showed differences between patients with acquired unilateral conductive hearing loss (UCHL) and those with congenital UCHL [8]. A factor that might play a role here is the onset of unilateral hearing loss. On average, patients with congenital UCHL experienced limited binaural hearing. The aim of this overview is to analyze the results of three studies performed in Nijmegen in more detail. In these studies, the patients were fitted with a BCD. Included in this overview are patients with acquired UCHL selected from Hol et al. [9], patients with congenital UCHL selected from Kunst et al. [10], and patients with bilateral hearing loss selected from Bosman et al. [11].

Measurements and Methods

Patients

Patients included in the original studies were selected according to the protocol described in the Baha (bone-anchored hearing aid) consensus paper [3]. For the present overview, the three patient groups are homogenized, and we added data of a group of normal-hearing controls. We excluded the 3 patients with mixed hearing loss (others had conductive hearing loss) from the study performed by Hol et al. [9]. Data of the children with UCHL were excluded from the study performed by Kunst et al. [10], and from the study performed by Bosman et al. [11] because of the different test protocol. Patients with congenital bilateral conductive hearing loss were excluded because of the limited group size and their slow progress in binaural performance [12]. Table 1 gives an overview of the number of patients and of the audiometric characteristics of the three patient groups that are compared. The patients comprised successive adult BCD users. Throughout the

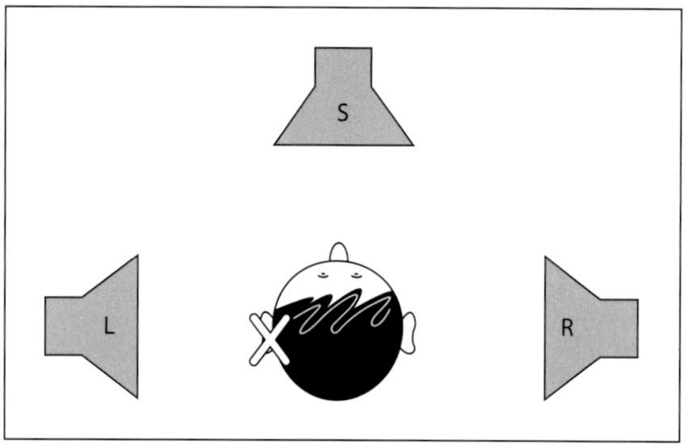

Fig. 1. Sound field setup with the loudspeaker S in front of the patient and the loudspeakers on the right (R at azimuth +90°) and on the left (L at azimuth –90°) side. The patient's left ear has conductive hearing loss, indicated by the cross. SRTs were measured while poor hearing was on the left (as depicted): head shadow = SRTul – SRTur, binaural advantage = SRTbr – SRTur, binaural disturbance = SRTbl – SRTul; when poor hearing was on the right: head shadow = SRTur – SRTul, binaural advantage = SRTbl – SRTul, binaural disturbance = SRTbr – SRTur. SRTul refers to measurement of the SRT with unilateral listening (u) and noise from the left (l). SRTbr refers to measurement of the SRT with bilateral listening (b) and noise from the right (r).

studies, the BCDs were fitted and evaluated by the same audiologists. All the BCDs (type Baha Classic or Baha Compact; Cochlear BAS, Gothenburg, Sweden) have linear amplification (not wide dynamic range compression) and omnidirectional microphones. Measurement protocols and equipment were the same in all patient groups.

For reference purposes, data were obtained from a control group of 10 subjects with normal hearing, who were listening with one ear plugged and covered with an ear muff (monaural), or with both ears open (binaural). Their headphone thresholds at 250 Hz to 8 kHz were 20 dB hearing loss or better for both ears. The plug and earmuff attenuated the sound with 30–40 dB.

Speech Perception

Speech perception was measured in the sound field using short, everyday Dutch sentences [13]. Speech reception thresholds (SRTs), the presentation level at which 50% of sentences were identified correctly, were established using an adaptive tracking procedure. SRTs were measured in quiet and in noise; in the latter case, steady-state noise was used with the same frequency spectrum as the long-term spectrum of the sentences [13]. Speech was presented by a loudspeaker in front of the patient (S), while the noise was presented by a loudspeaker on either the left (L) or right (R) of the patient (fig. 1). The noise level was fixed at 65 dBA in all the measurements. In each separate condition, the SRTs were measured twice and the results were averaged.

Figure 1 illustrates the measurement in a subject with poor hearing on the left side. This condition applies to the unaided situation in the UCHL patients, the unilateral BCD fitting in the bilateral patients and the condition with one ear blocked in the controls. Unilateral SRTs were determined with the noise coming from the left speaker and separately from the right speaker. Next, the measurements were repeated while listening with both ears, thus either (fully) aided or, in the case of the controls, with both ears open. The following outcomes were calculated when poor hearing was on the left (as presented in fig. 1): (a) Head shadow effect (HSE), which was defined as the unilateral SRTs with noise presented at left minus SRTs with noise presented at right. (b) The binaural advantage, which was defined as the bilateral SRT with noise at the right minus the unilateral SRT with noise at the right. (c) The binaural disturbance, which was defined as the bilateral SRT with noise at the left minus the unilateral SRT with noise at the left. (d) The binaural summation which was defined as the change in the SRT in quiet when listening unilaterally minus bilaterally. In the legends of figure 1, all possible calculations (also the calculations when poor hearing was on the right side) are listed.

The binaural disturbance score is expected to be zero when the listener can effectively disregard the input from a particular ear. If the score is positive, then the (second) BCD is causing disturbance instead of being helpful. In subjects with normal hearing, there might even be an improvement in this bilateral listening condition (thus score <0), because the noise heard in the left ear during bilateral listening is not in phase with the noise heard in the other ear. This so-called binaural squelch might then play a role. If the binaural advantage score is comparable with the head shadow score, then the head shadow has effectively been eliminated by the BCD. If the binaural advantage is smaller, then the BCD has only partially compensated for the head shadow. When it is larger, then binaural squelch is present.

Directional Hearing

Sound localization in the horizontal plane was studied with eleven loudspeakers in a circle (between –120 and 120°) at intervals of 30°. The radius of the circle was 1.2 m; the patient's head was at the centre of the circle. Stimuli consisted of one-second bursts of 1/3 octave band filtered noise, with either 500 or 3,000 Hz as the centre frequency. Stimuli were presented at 65 dB SPL, four times per loudspeaker in a random order, which resulted in 44 stimuli per measurement condition. After each stimulus, the patient was asked to indicate the loudspeaker that had produced the sound. Patients were not permitted to turn their head during stimulus presentation. No training or feedback was given. Per stimulus, the difference in azimuth was determined between the position of the loudspeaker that had produced the sound and the position of the loudspeaker that was indicated by the patient. Responses to stimuli presented with the two outermost loudspeakers, at +120° and –120°, were not included in the analysis. Mean absolute difference in azimuth, called the MAE (mean absolute error, in degrees) was the outcome measure. Computer simulation showed that the chance level of MAE was 73°. In the case of poor localization but good lateralization, the MAE score was approximately 35°.

All the tests were carried out in a sound-treated double-walled sound booth (reverberation time of 0.11 s), at least 10 weeks after the BCD had been fitted, to allow the patient time to adjust to the BCD.

Results

Speech Perception

Table 2 presents the mean results of the binaural hearing tests in the different subgroups.

Concerning the binaural summation scores, the best results were found in the patients with binaural hearing loss, whereas the poorest result, even a nonsignificant change, was found in the patients with congenital UCHL.

Differences in the HSE (data not presented in table) were found between the normal ears (4.4 ± 1.6 dB) and the hearing-impaired ears aided with a BCD (2.8 ± 2.1 dB). This was ascribed to the location of the BCD, outside the skull, a few cm behind and above the external auditory meatus. Thus, as the microphone of the BCD is positioned less effectively in the head shadow than the ear drum, on average, the (second) BCD can reduce the head shadow by only 2.8 dB.

In the control group, the binaural advantage (4.6 dB) was somewhat larger than the HSE (which was 4.4 dB), suggesting an additional squelch effect. However, this 0.2 dB difference was not statistically significant. Furthermore, the binaural disturbance score was not statistically different from zero; again, this means that there was no evidence of a squelch effect. In the bilateral patients and patients with acquired UCHL, the binaural advantage score was close to 2.8 dB, i.e. the head shadow maximally compensated with the BCD. This means that the BCD reduced the head shadow effectively; but again, no squelch effect was found. Results in the patients with congenital UCHL differed from those in the other groups: the head shadow was only partially compensated for by the BCD. In fact, on an individual level, the difference between the binaural advantage and the HSE was an average of 1.8 ± 2.2, which was significantly different from zero ($t = 2.59$; $p = 0.03$).

Directional Hearing

Table 3 presents the results of the directional hearing tests at 500 and 3,000 Hz. The subjects with normal hearing were first tested with one ear occluded. Mean MAE values were 64° at 500 Hz and 83° at 3,000 Hz (see table 3). This was near change level, which was 73°. With the occluded ear open again, mean MAEs improved to 8° at the two test frequencies. These data are considered to validate the measurement setup. They indicate MAEs <10° in cases of normal hearing. The data also indicate that the attenuation of the plug for low frequencies (500 Hz) was considerably less than for high frequencies (3,000 Hz) as the mean MAE values were slightly below change level at 500 Hz.

The data obtained from patients with bilateral hearing loss group were somewhat different. While listening with one BCD, their mean score was 66° at 500 Hz and 56° at 3,000 Hz, which was somewhat better than chance level. With the second BCD active, the MAE dropped significantly to a value of around 25° at the two test frequencies. In the patients with acquired UCHL, unaided scores were around 40–45°. In the aided condition, the MAE improved significantly to around 15°. In patients with congenital UCHL, the unaided MAE was 35–40°, thus fairly good. Obviously,

Table 2. Mean (SD) results from the speech perception test in dB

Group	Binaural advantage	Binaural disturbance	Binaural summation
Acquired UCHL	2.6 (1.7)**	0.2 (2.5)	2.2 (1.5)**
Congenital UCHL	1.1 (1.9)	0.4 (1.9)	1.3 (2.4)
Bilateral HL	2.5 (1.8)**	0.6 (1.5)	4.0 (3.1)**
Control listeners	4.6 (1.6)**	0.2 (1.2)	n.a.

**p < 0.05, two-sided t test; n.a. = not available.

Table 3. MAE (SD) in degrees in the different groups

Group	500 Hz NB noise		3,000 Hz NB noise	
	unilateral	bilateral	unilateral	bilateral
Acquired UCHL	46 (20)	12 (10)*	38 (21)	16 (12)*
Congenital UCHL	34 (24)	30 (13)	39 (30)	31 (18)
Bilateral HL	66 (14)	26 (8)*	56 (13)	25 (8)*
Control listeners	64 (14)	8 (7)*	83 (9)	8 (10)*

*p < 0.025, two-sided t test. NB = Narrow-band noise.

the congenital UCHL patients had acquired a certain level of directional hearing. In the congenital UCHL subgroup, remarkably, only a minor, nonsignificant improvement in MAE was found in the BCD-aided condition.

Table 3 shows that at the two frequencies, the aided MAE scores were fairly comparable within the subgroups. The significantly improved MAE values in patients with binaural hearing loss and acquired UCHL suggest that BCD application provided these patients with effective interaural time (phase) cues and interaural intensity cues. On average, BCD application was not beneficial in patients with congenital UCHL.

Discussion

Speech Perception in Quiet

Patients with bilateral hearing loss had the best binaural summation score (table 2). This score was well within the normal range (3–6 dB). In the patients with UCHL, binaural summation was less distinct. This might be ascribed to asymmetrical 'aided' hearing thresholds. In comparison with the normal ear, the BCD-aided thresholds were 10–15 dB poorer in the patients with acquired [9] and congenital [10] UCHL. In contrast, bilateral BCDs in the bilateral hearing loss group led to symmetrical hearing thresholds [11].

The low, nonsignificant summation score in the patients with congenital UCHL suggests either poor interaural interaction or disturbance in perception caused by cross-hearing. If so, the latter factor does not play a role in patients with acquired UCHL who had good binaural summation scores.

Speech Perception in Noise

In the control group, bilateral listening effectively eliminated the head shadow, but there was no evidence of binaural squelch in the present measurement setup. Bilateral listening effectively compensated for the head shadow for all the patient groups except for the patients with congenital UCHL. Only a minor part of their head shadow was compensated for. There was no significant binaural disturbance in any of the groups (column 2, table 2).

Directional Hearing: Monaural Listening Condition

Mean MAE in the unilateral listening condition was poor in all the groups, but not necessarily at chance level (see table 3, columns 1 and 3). It was better than chance level in the patients with UCHL: 34–46°. This is in accordance with the literature [14]. Patients with congenital UCHL had the best unaided MAE scores, which suggest that these patients had learned to cope with unilateral hearing somewhat better than the patients with acquired UCHL.

Directional Hearing: Bilateral Listening Condition

MAE scores improved significantly in patients with acquired UCHL when they were listening with their BCD turned on. Compared to the results in these patients, results were surprisingly poor with the BCD active in patients with congenital UCHL. The latter patients had not received the BCD until adulthood, which might be well past the *sensitive period for binaural hearing development* (as has been shown in animal research [15]). At an individual level, significant variance in the results of patients with congenital UCHL has been reported [10]. The performance of some of them was even better with than without the BCD, whereas others showed significant improvement in directional hearing [10]. Priwin et al. [16] reported similar results. This suggests that cross-hearing, i.e. stimulation of the contralateral cochlea during bone conduction, might cause disturbance in some patients with congenital UCHL. It should be noted that the presented results of the patients with congenital UCHL were obtained at reevaluations after at least 10 months of BCD use [10], which implies that any further improvement, because of learning, is unlikely.

The MAE scores in patients with bilateral hearing loss were much better in the bilateral-aided condition than in the unilateral condition, but still not below 25°. An explanation for the poor responses to the 500-Hz stimulus might be that the interaural time difference is a maximum of 0.2 ms with bone conduction stimulation, whereas in subjects with normal hearing, proper sound localization in the low frequencies requires a perceived interaural time difference of between 0 and 0.7 ms, depending on azimuth. A maximum interaural time difference of 0.2 ms might have a second disadvantage. In the case of bilateral stimulation via bone conduction, direct and delayed crossover stimulation might cause interference in a particular ear, with the largest effect at the high frequencies [17]. Such interferences will affect interaural loudness differences and thus directional hearing. The poor bilateral MAE scores in response to the 3,000 Hz might have been caused by such interference. Furthermore, the less effective acoustic separation by head shadow might have played a role.

In all the subgroups, the numbers of patients were limited. However, additional support for the present observations can be found in the BCD literature. Priwin et al. [18] performed a study on 12 patients with bilateral BCDs that was fairly similar to that of Bosman et al. [11]. They reported significantly improved directional hearing in the bilateral BCD condition and a summation effect of 5.4 dB (Bosman: 4.0 dB). Based on their data, the binaural advantage score was calculated as 3.1 dB (Bosman: 2.5 dB) and the binaural disturbance score as 1 dB (Bosman: 0.6 dB). Thus, their data showed the same trends as those reported by Bosman et al. [11].

Patients with congenital UCHL comprised the 10 adults from the group of 20 patients studied by Kunst et al. [10]. The other 10 patients were children, fitted with the BCD between age 5 and 14 years. They were evaluated using comparable but more child-friendly tests. The children's directional hearing and speech perception in noise results showed the same trends as those in the adults, namely the large variation in the results and the observation that the performance of some of the children was even better without than with the BCD, which supports the conclusions drawn from the adult data [10]. Priwin et al. [17] reported similar poor results in children with congenital UCHL. Indeed, animal research indicated that there are differences in the neuronal processing of sound between animals with congenital and acquired UCHL. It has been demonstrated that induced UCHL resulted in reduced neuronal size in neonatal animals [19], while it did not affect neuronal size in older animals [20].

Conclusions

Bilateral BCD application was beneficial to the patients with bilateral conductive or mixed hearing loss. Nevertheless, the results were somewhat poorer than those obtained from subjects with normal hearing. Good results were also found in the patients with acquired UCHL fitted with a BCD, but not in the patients with congenital UCHL. More research is needed to fully understand these observations, notably the influence of cross-hearing and the HSE and to determine the sensitive period for the development of binaural hearing.

References

1 Hausler R, Colburn S, Marr E: Sound localization in subjects with impaired hearing. Acta Otolaryngol (Stockh) 1983;400(suppl):5–62.
2 Mylanus EAM, Van der Pouw KC, Snik AFM, Cremers CWRJ: Intraindividual comparison of the bone-anchored hearing aid and air-conduction hearing aids. Arch Otolaryngol Head Neck Surg 1998;124:271–276.
3 Snik AFM, Mylanus EAM, Proops DW, Wolfaardt JF, Hodgetts WE, Somers T, Niparko JK, Wazen JJ, Sterkers O, Cremers CWRJ, Tjellström A: Consensus statements on the BAHA system: where do we stand at present? Ann Otol Rhinol Laryngol 2005;195(suppl):2–12.
4 Stenfelt S, Goode RL: Bone-conducted sound: physiological and clinical aspects. Otol Neurotol 2005;26:1245–1261.
5 Stenfelt S: Bilateral fitting of BAHAs and BAHA fitted in unilateral deaf persons: acoustical aspects. Int J Audiol 2005;44: 178–189.
6 Kaga K, Setou M, Nakamura M: Bone-conducted sound lateralization of interaural time difference and interaural intensity difference in children and young adults with bilateral microtia and atresia of the ears. Acta Otolaryngol 2001;121:274–277.
7 MacDonald JA, Henry PP, Letowski TR: Spatial audio through a bone conduction interface. Int J Audiol 2006;45:595–599.
8 Snik AFM, Mylanus EAM, Cremers CWRJ: The bone-anchored hearing aid in patients with a unilateral air-bone gap. Otol Neurotol 2002;23:61–66.
9 Hol MKS, Snik AFM, Mylanus EAM, Cremers CWRJ: Does the bone-anchored hearing aid have a complementary effect on audiological and subjective outcomes in patients with unilateral conductive hearing loss? Audiol Neurootol 2005;10: 159–168.
10 Kunst SJW, Leijendeckers JM, Mylanus EAM, Hol MKS, Snik AFM, Cremers CWRJ: Bone-anchored hearing aid system application for unilateral congenital conductive hearing impairment: audiometric results. Otol Neurotol 2008;29:2–7.
11 Bosman AJ, Snik AFM, Van der Pouw CTM, Mylanus EAM, Cremers CWRJ: Audiometric evaluation of bilaterally fitted bone-anchored hearing aids. Audiol 2001;40:158–167.
12 Van der Pouw CTM, Snik AFM, Cremers CWRJ: Audiometric results of bilateral bone-anchored hearing aid application with bilateral congenital aural atresia. Laryngoscope 1998;108:548–553.
13 Plomp R, Mimpen AM: Improving the reliability of testing the speech reception threshold for sentences. Audiology 1979; 18:43–52.

14 Wright BA, Zhang Y: A review of learning with normal and altered sound-localization cues in human adults. Int J Audiol 2006;45(suppl):592–598.
15 King AJ, Parsons CH, Moore DR: Plasticity in the neural coding of auditory space in the mammalian brain. Proc Nat Acad Sci USA 2000;97:11821–11828.
16 Priwin C, Stenfelt S, Granström G, Tjellström A, Håkansson B: Bilateral bone-anchored hearing aids (BAHAs): an audiometric evaluation. Laryngoscope 2004;114:77–84.
17 Rowan D, Gray M: Lateralization of high-frequency pure tones with interaural phase difference and bone conduction. Int J Audiol 2008;47:404–411.
18 Priwin C, Jönsson R, Hultcrantz M, Granström G: BAHA in children and adolescents with unilateral or bilateral conductive hearing loss: a study of outcome. Int J Pediatr Otorhinolaryngol 2007;71:135–145.
19 Webster DB: Auditory neuronal size after a unilateral conductive hearing loss. Exp Neurol 1983;79:130–140.
20 Webster DB: Late onset of auditory deprivation does not affect brain stem auditory neuron soma size. Hear Res 1983;12:145–147.

A. Snik
Department of Otorhinolaryngology, Radboud University Medical Centre
PO Box 9101
6500 HB Nijmegen (The Netherlands)
Tel. +31 24 3610397, Fax +31 24 3540251, E-Mail a.snik@kno.umcn.nl

Kompis M, Caversaccio M-D (eds): Implantable Bone Conduction Hearing Aids.
Adv Otorhinolaryngol. Basel, Karger, 2011, vol 71, pp 92–102

Bone-Anchored Devices in Single-Sided Deafness

C.M. Stewart · J.H. Clark · J.K. Niparko

Department of Otolaryngology-Head and Neck Surgery, Johns Hopkins School of Medicine, Baltimore, Md., USA

Abstract

Single-sided deafness (SSD) implies sensorineural hearing loss in one ear with normal contralateral hearing function. Traditionally, SSD patients have been overlooked due to a belief that the preserved functioning of the contralateral ear compensates for the nonhearing side. SSD patients however experience multiple audiological difficulties, particularly when the sound source is situated on the non-hearing side or in the presence of competing sounds. Through reviewing current literature, we describe the role of bone-anchored devices (Baha) in the management of SSD patients. Recent publications for Baha in SSD have demonstrated consistent objective and subjective improvement in audiologic metrics when compared to unaided conditions. There is also evidence of benefit provided by Baha by the Abbreviated Profile of Hearing Aid Benefit, in global measures of ease of communication, reverberation, and background noise, but not typically in aversiveness to sounds. Interestingly, despite some patients gaining minimal objective or subjective benefits, the majority of these patients still report improved quality of life and would recommend the procedure. Despite increasing evidence for the role of Baha in the management of SSD in the literature, much of these data are based on older technology. Further reports should specify the processor type used and the etiology of the hearing loss to ensure accuracy of future data.

Bone-anchored hearing devices (Baha) have been used for surgical restoration of hearing loss since 1977, and are currently used for a variety of unilateral and bilateral hearing loss categories including conductive hearing loss, mixed hearing loss, and profound unilateral sensorineural hearing loss, referred to here as single-sided deafness (SSD). Interval development of external processors with increasing power and digital signal processing sophistication has led to a corresponding evolution in outcomes after surgery over time. In addition, there are now multiple processors and Baha prostheses available from two manufacturers (Baha from Cochelar Americas, Inc., Centennial, Colo., USA, and Ponto from Oticon USA, Inc., Somerset, N.J., USA). Figure 1 shows the new BP-100 device from Cochlear Corporation. This review focuses on the audiologic aspects of Baha in SSD [for recent comprehensive review, see 1]; other types of hearing loss and Baha are discussed elsewhere in this volume.

The Baha operates via technologies and mechanisms that are distinctly different from those utilized by both air- and bone-conducting conventional hearing aids. The system uniquely utilizes bone transmission to stimulate the cochlea through an implant that requires surgical placement. Device selection is contingent on medical

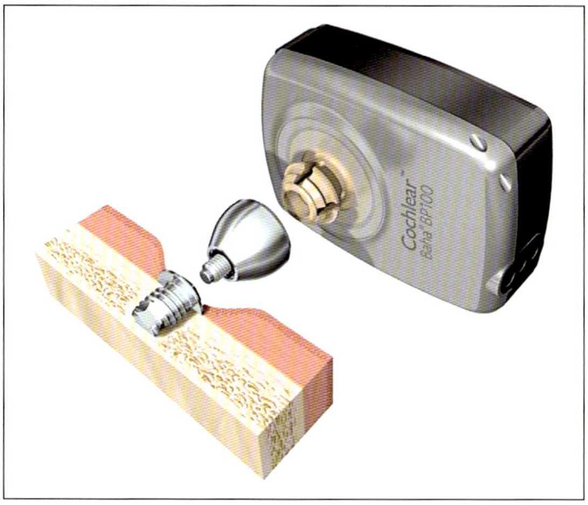

Fig. 1. The new BP-100 device from Cochlear Corporation. Copyright Cochlear Corporation.

necessity as judged by a physician who must consider other treatment alternatives, and surgically implant the device if a BAHA treatment strategy is deemed necessary. The US Centers for Medicaid & Medicare Services identifies the Baha system as distinctly classified as a *device* (osseointegrated implant) and not a hearing aid [2].

SSD implies normal contralateral hearing, defined as pure tone average ≤20 measured at 0.5, 1, 2, and 3 kHz. Common causes of SSD include acoustic neuroma (untreated, treated with surgery or radiotherapy), sudden sensorineural hearing loss, congenital hearing loss, and Ménière's disease. The majority of Baha for SSD combine these groups, and utilize multiple, external processors. See table 1 for summary of sample size, etiology and audiologic metrics utilized in the studies described for the literature review [3–10] of the role of Baha in the management of SSD.

The benefits of binaural hearing are gained through the ability to utilize loudness summation, and sound localization, whilst eliminating head shadow effect, optimizing both speech intelligibility in noise and spatial balance [11, 12]. Despite individuals with SSD having functional hearing sufficient to acquire speech, language, education and vocational skills, they typically experience difficulties in verbal communication under certain circumstances where these benefits of binaural hearing become apparent [13, 14]. As a result, individuals with SSD have difficulty in listening environments where the sound source of interest is either positioned on the side of impairment or when reverberations, background noise or an unfamiliar speaker corrupt the cues for sound localization [14, 15]. Figure 2 demonstrates Baha placement and fitting for right SSD.

Sound on the Side of Impairment/Head Shadow

The role of the head in diffracting sound, or head shadow effect, is well established [16], and pertains to the way sound is altered by obstacles it encounters. Obstacles larger than the sound wave prevent the passing of that sound, resulting in a shadowing effect on the contralateral side of the obstacle whilst causing an increased sound pressure on the ipsilateral side to the sound source [17]. This effect is therefore more pronounced at high frequencies (and shorter wavelengths), with a sound signal on the nonhearing side being attenuated by 10–16 dB above 1,000 Hz by the time it reaches the good ear in an individual with SSD [11, 18].

Conventional Solutions

SSD has traditionally been a largely neglected and ignored audiological entity by the medical community with some affected individuals being simply advised to sit close and turn the better-hearing ear towards the sound source [19]. Newman et al. [20] investigated the perceived hearing handicap in individuals with unilateral or mild hearing loss, and found that patients encountered a number of emotional and social-situational problems. They also found great variation in the individual's reaction

Table 1. Summary of sample size, etiology and audiologic metrics utilized in the studies described for the literature review of the role of Baha in the management of SSD

Article number	Authors	Total	AN	SSHL	MD	Congenital	Other	Audiologic metrics
1	Martin et al. [3]	58	27	9	0	7	15	Speech in noise
								GBI
								SSQ
2	Gluth et al. [4]	21	5	6	4	1	5	Glasgow hearing aid benefit profile
								APHAB
								Single-Sided Deafness Questionnaire
3	Schrøder et al. [5]	21	15	1	1	0	4	Custom Questionnaire
4	Wazen et al. [6]	21	unknown	unknown	unknown	unknown	unknown	Pure tone air and bone
								NU-6
								CNC
								HINT
								Hearing Satisfaction Scale
								Baha Comparison Questionnaire
								GBI
5	Christensen et al. [7]	23	unknown	unknown	unknown	unknown	unknown	HINT
								Children's Home Inventory for Listening Difficulties
6	Hol et al. [8]	10	1	2	0	2	4	APHAB
								SSQ
								Single-Sided Deafness Questionnaire
7	Yuen et al. [9]	21	9	3	1	1	7	APHAB
								Glasgow hearing aid benefit profile
								HINT

Table 1. Continued

Article number	Authors	Total	AN	SSHL	MD	Congenital	Other	Audiologic metrics
8	Dumper et al. [10]	50	unknown	unknown	unknown	unknown	unknown	HINT
		15 BCHL						APHAB
		10 UCHL						SSQ
		10 UMHL						
		15 SSD						

AN = Acoustic neuroma; SSHL = sudden sensorineural hearing loss; MD = Ménière's disease; BCHL = bilateral conductive hearing loss; UCHL = unilateral conductive hearing loss; UMHL = unilateral mixed hearing loss.

to their own hearing loss, and concluded that perceived communication and psychosocial handicap cannot be determined from an audiogram, which highlights the importance of assessing individuals with unilateral or mild hearing loss.

A number of treatment modalities are available:

Contralateral Routing of Signal Aid

Contralateral Routing of Signal (CROS) aid is a device consisting of two parts, a microphone which is worn on the deaf side and a hearing aid which is worn in the good ear. The two parts are connected either by wire or infrared/radio frequency, and sound is transmitted from the microphone to the hearing aid in an attempt to eliminate head shadow. However, the results gained with CROS hearing aids have been disappointing, with common complaints of social stigma related to poor cosmesis, discomfort and overall poor hearing gains [1]. Hill et al. [19] investigated satisfaction with digital CROS and bilateral CROS hearing aids and found greater satisfaction with the new generation digital devices compared to older analog hearing aids. In addition to improved hearing outcome achieved with digital devices, the authors attributed appropriate candidate selection, proper fitting, and close follow-up of recipients for the higher level of satisfaction.

Conventional Hearing Aid

A conventional air conduction hearing aid may be used on the deaf side, and provide transcranial stimulation without the necessary occlusion of the hearing ear as in CROS. This requires significant power, and a deeper, more medial ear mold of a completely in the canal (CIC) hearing aid [21]. A recent study randomized the order of use for conventional CROS, CIC, and headband BAHA; CIC demonstrated objective and subjective benefit; however, of the 10 patients none selected CIC, 1 selected CROS, 3 selected Baha surgery, and 6 chose no further rehabilitation [8].

Role of Baha

Surgical rehabilitation of SSD with Baha was first reported in 2000 and 2001 by Vaneecloo et al. [22, 23], and approved by the United States Food and Drug Administration (FDA) in 2002. Worldwide application of Baha for SSD is likely related to the earlier, overwhelming success of Baha for the earlier indications of conductive

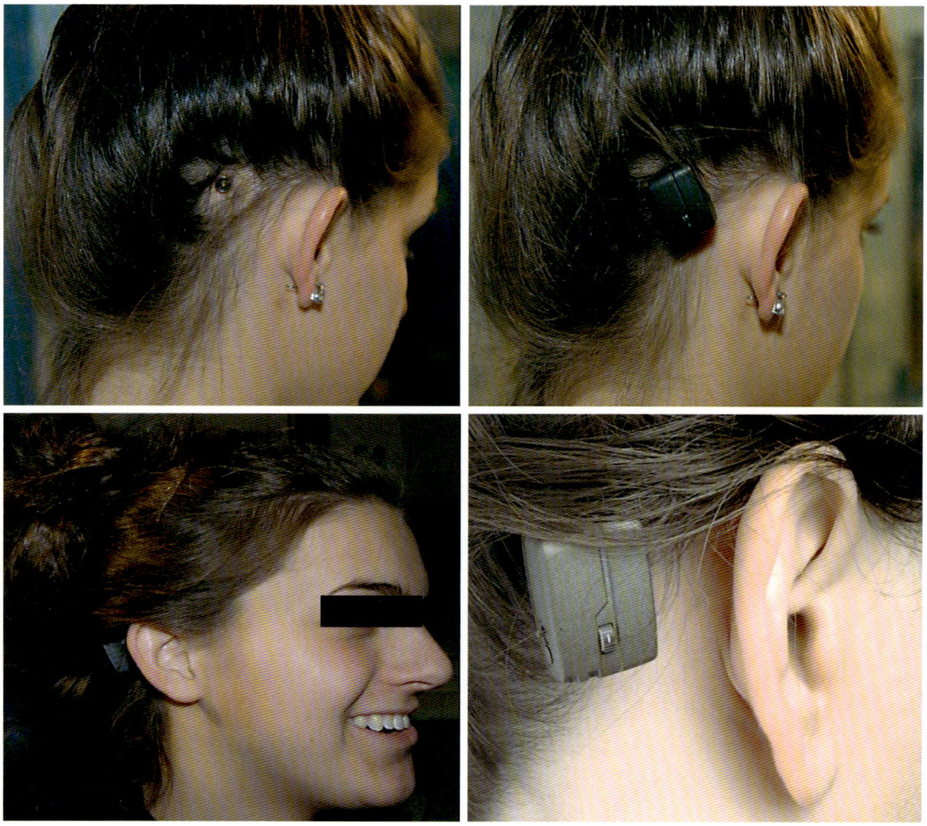

Fig. 2. Baha placement and fitting for right SSD.

hearing loss, and mixed hearing loss. Preliminary studies, retrospective studies, and controlled trials have demonstrated some subjective and objective benefits when compared to unaided and other aided (notably CROS) conditions, see table 1 and discussion below. Inherent in interpretation of these efforts are the basic questions of how to assess the audiologic handicap of SSD, and how to assess the benefits of surgical rehabilitation of SSD by Baha.

SSD Handicap

The Speech, Spatial, and Qualities of Hearing Questionnaire (SSQ) was developed in 2004 [24]. This pioneering instrument uses a 10-point scale to investigate areas of communication and hearing absent or underrepresented in earlier hearing aid evaluation instruments [for review of Dr Gatehouse's legacy, see 25]. The speech component queries speech understanding using 14 scenarios of speech conversation or listening in a variety of challenging and real-life situations such as multiple speakers, speech in noise, listening to the television, radio, or telephone. The spatial component investigates sound awareness in space with 17 scenarios such as speaker identification, direction of familiar or unfamiliar sounds, and the speed and direction of moving sounds. The quality component uses 18 scenarios to assess sound and speech perception as natural, recognizable or

Table 2. The SSQ – subsets with visual analog scale, and representative sample scenarios for each component [25]

SPEECH			
You are in a group of about five people, sitting round a table. It is an otherwise quiet place. You can see everyone else in the group. Can you follow the conversation?	Min (Not at all)	0 1 2 3 4 5 6 7 8 9 10	Max (Perfect)
Can you have a conversation with someone when another person is speaking whose voice is the same pitch as the person you're talking to?	Min (Not at all)	0 1 2 3 4 5 6 7 8 9 10	Max (Perfect)
Can you have a conversation with someone when another person is speaking whose voice is different in pitch from the person you're talking to?	Min (Not at all)	0 1 2 3 4 5 6 7 8 9 10	Max (Perfect)
You are in conversation with one person in a room where there are many other people talking. Can you follow what the person you are talking to is saying?	Min (Not at all)	0 1 2 3 4 5 6 7 8 9 10	Max (Perfect)
You are with a group and the conversation switches from one person to another. Can you easily follow the conversation without missing the start of what each new speaker is saying?	Min (Not at all)	0 1 2 3 4 5 6 7 8 9 10	Max (Perfect)
SPATIAL			
You are outdoors in an unfamiliar place. You hear someone using a lawnmower. You can't see where they are. Can you tell right away where the sound is coming from?	Min (Not at all)	0 1 2 3 4 5 6 7 8 9 10	Max (Perfect)
You are in the stairwell of a building with floors above and below you. You can hear sounds from another floor. Can you readily tell where the sound is coming from?	Min (Not at all)	0 1 2 3 4 5 6 7 8 9 10	Max (Perfect)

Table 2. Continued

SPATIAL			
You are standing on the footpath of a busy street. Can you hear right away which direction a bus or truck is coming from before you see it?	Min (Not at all)	0 1 2 3 4 5 6 7 8 9 10	Max (Perfect)
Can you tell from their voice or footsteps whether the person is coming towards you or going away?	Min (Not at all)	0 1 2 3 4 5 6 7 8 9 10	Max (Perfect)
Do you have the impression of sounds being exactly where you would expect them to be?	Min (Not at all)	0 1 2 3 4 5 6 7 8 9 10	Max (Perfect)
QUALITIES			
You are in a room and there is music on the radio. Someone else in the room is talking. Can you hear the voice as something separate from the music?	Min (Not at all)	0 1 2 3 4 5 6 7 8 9 10	Max (Perfect)
Do you find it easy to distinguish different pieces of music that you are familiar with?	Min (Not at all)	0 1 2 3 4 5 6 7 8 9 10	Max (Perfect)
Can you tell the difference between different sounds, for example, a car versus a bus; water boiling in a pot versus food cooking in a frying pan?	Min (Not at all)	0 1 2 3 4 5 6 7 8 9 10	Max (Perfect)
Do other people's voices sound clear and natural?	Min (Not at all)	0 1 2 3 4 5 6 7 8 9 10	Max (Perfect)
When you are a passenger can you easily hear what the driver is saying sitting alongside you?	Min (Not at all)	0 1 2 3 4 5 6 7 8 9 10	Max (Perfect)

distinct. See table 2 for representative questions and the 10-point visual analog scale. The SSQ instrument was used to assess the subjective disability of SSD patients after surgical treatment of acoustic neuroma [26]. This study characterizes the significant auditory handicap associated with SSD when the specifics of speech, sound in space, and sound quality are considered; see figure 1 of this study in particular. These data demonstrate the significant perceived handicap for SSD after surgery for AN. There are significant differences in nearly every domain when compared to age and hearing (better hearing ear)-matched controls. This study clearly demonstrates the ability of the SSQ to discriminate the subjective handicap of SSD. The SSQ Handicap questionnaire was preceded by the SSD questionnaire published in 2003 [11] and occasionally used [27, 28].

The Glasgow Hearing Aid Benefit Profile (GHABP) is a validated measure of individual benefit after fitting and use of hearing aid or Baha [29]. Specific domains include satisfaction, use, benefit, and initial and subsequent disability. The Abbreviated Profile of Hearing Aid Benefit (APHAB) is another instrument that examines multiple domains of hearing [30]. These four domains include hearing in background noise, reverberant conditions, ease of communication, and aversiveness to sound. The Glasgow Benefit Inventory (GBI) is another innovative instrument developed by Dr. Gatehouse and colleagues [31] that measures benefit after intervention. The GBI has occasionally been used to assess Baha outcomes [3, 32, 33]. The use of these various instruments relating the Baha and SSD are summarized in table 1.

Literature Overview

Relative benefits of Baha versus CROS in SSD were the subject of a meta-analysis in 2006 [21], updated by the authors in 2009 [34]. In addition, this topic was reviewed as part of an extensive review of SSD this year [1]. When outcomes were assessed with APHAB, domains consistently superior with Baha included background noise, reverberant conditions, and aversiveness to sound, with no significant difference in ease of communication. As noted by Baguley et al. [34], the number of patients is relatively low. In addition, there are variations in subjects and technologies. Some older studies necessarily compare analog CROS devices with Baha technologies that are no longer available. Many of the important points addressed by Baguley et al. [34] have recently been addressed by Hol et al. [8]. In this prospective, randomized study, 10 SSD subjects each had 8-week trials for three different modes of rehabilitation, with the order or therapy randomized. The three modes were CROS (Widex B2 matched with WIDEX CROS), CIC (Belton, deep mould, maximal gain), and Baha on a headband (processor not stated). Outcomes evaluated included speech in noise testing, localization, and the APHAB, SSQ, and SSD questionnaire instruments. All three modes were subjectively and objectively better than the unaided condition. CROS performance across APHAB was generally best. The CIC was worse than unaided except in reverberant conditions. Reported SSQ data were limited to the spatial domain, which showed improvement over unaided, and similar values between modes (unaided mean 3.7, CROS mean 5.0, CIC mean 4.0, and headband Baha 4.8). The authors note that for such a trial the Baha headband is required since none of the patients has been implanted; as such, this Baha trial is a bone-conducted hearing aid, not a bone-anchored device.

The results of Baha for 58 patients with SSD were reported by Martin et al. [3]. This retrospective study used SSD as controls, and the cases were fit with Divino (16) or Compact (38) processors. Outcomes included speech in noise testing, SSQ, and GBI. Speech in noise testing was performed in 19 patients, with decreased speech discrimination with noise to the front and Baha side, and increased discrimination with speech in front and noise to the non-Baha side. The SSQ instrument was completed by 46 patients, and was remarkable for no difference between case and controls for any domain of speech, spatial, or quality rating. The GBI instrument was completed by 42 patients, with 14 reporting Benefit scores of ≤0, with a median value of +11 (means not reported), with greater Benefit scores (+15) for patients with SSD >10 years compared with +5 for SSD <10 years.

Long-term and short-term benefits were examined by a prospective study published by Gluth et al. [4]. This group of 21 patients was fit with Compact (15) and Divino (6) processors. Comparison of preoperative APHAB with long-term postoperative APHAB are significantly different over all domains ($p = 0.001$), but not for the individual domains ease of communication ($p = 0.079$) or aversiveness to sound ($p = 0.460$). GHABP demonstrated significant decrease in disability over nearly all measures. SSD questionnaire results demonstrated high rates of improvement in quality of life (69%), and long-term usage (85% >5 days/week). Schrøder et al. [5] reported similar subjective improvement using a custom questionnaire in a cohort of 21 patients.

Wazen et al. [6] reported the first audiologic results of 21 patients with SSD and Baha in patients fitted with the Intenso processor. Each patient was tested without Baha (unaided), with the Divino processor, and after a 4-week acclimatization period, with the Intenso processor. Audiologic testing included air and bone pure tone thresholds, and sound field testing with consonant nucleus consonant (CNC), Northwestern University Auditory Test 6 (NU-6), and Hearing in Noise Test (HINT). Subjective measures included the GBI and questionnaires about hearing satisfaction and device comparison. NU-6, CNC, and HINT were all significantly improved comparing Baha (Intenso and Divino) with unaided (see Wazen et al. [6] and fig. 1 for more details). Comparisons between Intenso and Divino were not significantly different. GBI scores for improved quality of life were +21, with 91% of patients saying they would recommend Baha to others. Patients who preferred a device preferred Intenso 4:1; 45% had no preference. The audiologic differences between Intenso and other processors were examined by Bosman et al. [35]. In this study, 23 patients were tested with their originally fitted Baha processor [Classic (11), Cordelle (4), or Compact (8)] versus Intenso. Thirty-five percent preferred their own processor over the Intenso. Signal-to-noise ratio performance was lowered (indicating increased speech discrimination) for Intenso versus own Baha, and APHAB scores lower (indicating decreased disability) for all domains except aversiveness to sound.

Christensen et al. [7] reported results in 23 children with SSD treated with Baha (Intenso or Divino). Average HINT score percentages improved at all signal to noise ratios: at 0 dB children younger than 13 years improved from 34 to 75% correct, teenagers improved from 33 to 87%.

Yuen et al. [9] described objective and subjective improvement in 21 patients with SSD treated with Baha [Compact (2), and Divino (19)]. HINT testing with speech applied to the Baha side and noise to the hearing side led to significant differences between aided and unaided corresponding to approximately –6 dB signal-to-noise ratio (theoretically 10% increase correct for each –1 dB). Subjective benefits were assessed with the APHAB instrument. Significantly lower scores (indicating decreased disability) were noted for all domains except aversiveness to sound. Dumper et al. [10] studied 15 patients with SSD, with similar decreases in signal-to-noise ratio for noise to the hearing ear, and APHAB with increased benefit across all domains except aversiveness to sound.

Conclusions

Recent publications for Baha in SSD have demonstrated consistent objective and subjective improvement in audiologic metrics when compared to unaided conditions. The subjective handicap associated with SSD has been delineated with the SSQ instrument, and is nicely illustrated in figure 1 of Douglas et al. [26]. Compelling evidence for benefit is also provided by APHAB, especially the global measures of ease of communication, reverberation, and background noise, but typically not aversiveness to sounds. The SSD questionnaire question 3 (Has your quality of life improved?) and GBI (general questions) are also revealing. Despite objective or subjective benefits that appear to be minimally beneficial, the majority of patients describe improved quality of life and would recommend the procedure.

Recent reports continue to present data from older technology, often mentioning the processor type. It will be crucial for further reports to specify the processor types, as well as the etiology of hearing loss. In addition, we recommend clearly specifying the laterality of stimulation with respect to the Baha side: notations of left and right should be converted to ipsilesional and contralesional for clarity.

References

1 Bishop CE, Eby TL: The current status of audiologic rehabilitation for profound unilateral sensorineural hearing loss. Laryngoscope 2010;120:552–556.
2 Medicare Benefit Policy Manual. https://www.cms.gov/manuals/Downloads/bp102c16.pdf. Accessed January 15, 2011.
3 Martin TPC, Lowther R, Cooper H, Holder RL, Irving RM, Reid AP, Proops DW: The bone-anchored hearing aid in the rehabilitation of single-sided deafness: experience with 58 patients. Clin Otolaryngol 2010;35:284–290.
4 Gluth MB, Eager KM, Eikelboom RH, Atlas MD: Long-term benefit perception, complications, and device malfunction rate of bone-anchored hearing aid implantation for profound unilateral sensorineural hearing loss. Otol Neurotol 2010 Aug 20. [Epub ahead of print]
5 Schrøder SA, Ravn T, Bonding P: BAHA in single-sided deafness: patient compliance and subjective benefit. Otol Neurotol 2010;31:404–408.
6 Wazen JJ, Van Ess MJ, Alameda J, Ortega C, Modisett M, Pinsky K: The Baha system in patients with single-sided deafness and contralateral hearing loss. Otolaryngol Head Neck Surg 2010;142:554–559.
7 Christensen L, Richter GT, Dornhoffer JL: Update on bone-anchored hearing aids in pediatric patients with profound unilateral sensorineural hearing loss. Arch Otolaryngol Head Neck Surg 2010;136:175–177.
8 Hol MK, Kunst SJ, Snik AF, Cremers CW: Pilot study on the effectiveness of the conventional CROS, the transcranial CROS and the BAHA transcranial CROS in adults with unilateral inner ear deafness. Eur Arch Otorhinolaryngol 2010;267:889–896.
9 Yuen HW, Bodmer D, Smilsky K, Nedzelski JM, Chen JM: Management of single-sided deafness with the bone-anchored hearing aid. Otolaryngol Head Neck Surg 2009;141:16–23.
10 Dumper J, Hodgetts B, Liu R, Brandner N: Indications for bone-anchored hearing AIDS: a functional outcomes study. J Otolaryngol Head Neck Surg 2009;38:96–105.
11 Wazen JJ, Spitzer JB, Ghossaini SN, Fayad JN, Niparko JK, Cox K, Brackmann DE, Soli SD: Transcranial contralateral cochlear stimulation in unilateral deafness. Otolaryngol Head Neck Surg 2003;129:248–254.
12 Roland PS, Marple BF: Disorders of inner ear, eighth nerve, and CNS; in Roland PS, Marple BF, Meyerhoff WL (eds). Hearing Loss, New York, Thimer Medical Publisher, 1997, p 227.
13 Katz J Handbook of Clinical Audiology, 4th edition, Baltimore: Williams & Wilkins, 1994, p 611.
14 Lin LM, Bowditch S, Anderson MJ, May B, Cox KM, Niparko JK: Amplification in the rehabilitation of unilateral deafness: speech in noise and directional hearing effects with bone-anchored hearing and contralateral routing of signal amplification. Otol Neurotol 2006;27:172–182.
15 Plomp R: Binaural and monaural speech intelligibility of connected discourse in reverberation as a function of azimuth of a single competing sound source (speck or noise). Acustica 1976;34:300–311.
16 Byrne D: Some Implications of body baffle for hearing aid selection. Sound 1972;6:86–91.
17 Dillion H: Hearing Aids. New York, Thieme, 2001, p 6.
18 Festen JM, Plomp R: Speech-reception threshold in noise with one and two hearing aids. J Acoust Soc Am 1986;79:465–471.
19 Hill SL 3rd, Marcus A, Digges EN, Gillman N, Silverstein H: Assessment of patient satisfaction with various configurations of digital CROS and BiCROS hearing aids. Ear Nose Throat J 2006;85:427–430, 442.
20 Newman CW, Jacobson GP, Hug GA, Sandridge SA: Perceived hearing handicap of patients with unilateral or mild hearing loss. Ann Otol Rhinol Laryngol 1997;106:210–214.
21 Baguley DM, Bird J, Humphriss RL, Prevost AT: The evidence base for the application of contralateral bone anchored hearing aids in acquired unilateral sensorineural hearing loss in adults. Clin Otolaryngol 2006;31:6–14.
22 Vaneecloo FM, Hanson JN, Laroche C, Vincent C, Dehaussy J: Prosthetic rehabilitation of unilateral anakusis. Study with stereoaudiometry (in French). Ann Otolaryngol Chir Cervicofac 2000;117:410–417.

23 Vaneecloo FM, Ruzza I, Hanson JN, Gérard T, Dehaussy J, Cory M, Arrouet C, Vincent C: The monaural pseudo-stereophonic hearing aid (BAHA) in unilateral total deafness: a study of 29 patients (in French). Rev Laryngol Otol Rhinol (Bord) 2001;122:343–350.
24 Gatehouse S, Noble W: The Speech, Spatial and Qualities of Hearing Scale (SSQ). Int J Audiol 2004;43:85–99.
25 Akeroyd MA: Stuart Gatehouse: a brief life. Trends Amplif 2008;12:67–75.
26 Douglas SA, Yeung P, Daudia A, Gatehouse S, O'Donoghue GM: Spatial hearing disability after acoustic neuroma removal. Laryngoscope 2007; 117:1648–1651.
27 Linstrom CJ, Silverman CA, Yu GP: Efficacy of the bone-anchored hearing aid for single-sided deafness. Laryngoscope 2009;119:713–720.
28 Newman CW, Sandridge SA, Wodzisz LM: Longitudinal benefit from and satisfaction with the Baha system for patients with acquired unilateral sensorineural hearing loss. Otol Neurotol 2008;29:1123–1131.
29 Gatehouse S: A self-report outcome measure for the evaluation of hearing aid fittings and services. Health Bull (Edinb) 1999;57:424–436.
30 Cox RM, Alexander GC: The abbreviated profile of hearing aid benefit. Ear Hear 1995;16:176–186.
31 Robinson K, Gatehouse S, Browning GG: Measuring patient benefit from otorhinolaryngological surgery and therapy. Ann Otol Rhinol Laryngol 1996;105:415–422.
32 Dutt SN, McDermott AL, Jelbert A, Reid AP, Proops DW: The Glasgow benefit inventory in the evaluation of patient satisfaction with the bone-anchored hearing aid: quality of life issues. J Laryngol Otol Suppl 2002;28(suppl):7–14.
33 McLarnon CM, Davison T, Johnson IJ: Bone-anchored hearing aid: comparison of benefit by patient subgroups. Laryngoscope 2004;114:942–944.
34 Baguley DM, Plydoropulou V, Prevost AT: Bone anchored hearing aids for single-sided deafness. Clin Otolaryngol 2009;34:176–177.
35 Bosman AJ, Snik FM, Mylanus EA, Cremers WR: Fitting range of the BAHA Intenso. Int J Audiol 2009;48:346–352.

Dr. John K. Niparko, MD
Department of Otolaryngology-HNS, Johns Hopkins Outpatient Center
601 N. Caroline St.
Baltimore, MD 21287 (USA)
Tel. +1 410 955 2689, Fax +1 410 614 9444, E-Mail jnipark1@jhmi.edu

Kompis M, Caversaccio M-D (eds): Implantable Bone Conduction Hearing Aids.
Adv Otorhinolaryngol. Basel, Karger, 2011, vol 71, pp 103–111

Factors Influencing the Decision for Baha in Unilateral Deafness: The Bern Benefit in Single-Sided Deafness Questionnaire

Martin Kompis · Flurin Pfiffner · Martin Krebs · Marco-Domenico Caversaccio

Department of ENT, Head and Neck Surgery, Inselspital, University of Bern, Bern, Switzerland

Abstract

The data of 46 adults with single-sided sensorineural deafness who were candidates for bone-anchored hearing aids (Baha) CROS (contralateral routing of signals) were analyzed. All candidates tested a Baha with a headband in their normal environment. Subsequently, 29 of the candidates chose a permanent Baha CROS fitting, and 17 declined, thus forming the two study groups. No significant difference regarding age, sex or duration of deafness was found between the two groups. Similarly, the transcranial attenuation was not significantly different between those who accepted and declined a Baha. Subjects with some residual hearing in their poorer ear tended to decline a Baha, but the effect was not statistically significant. For a subset of 28 subjects, the Bern Benefit in Single-Sided Deafness questionnaire was administered. The questionnaire consists of 10 visual analogue scales rating the subjectively perceived benefit of the Baha or any other CROS device in different situations. Scores were found to be significantly higher for speech understanding at some distance ($p = 0.026$), for speech understanding in noise ($p = 0.037$), for group conversations ($p < 0.01$), and for the overall benefit ($p < 0.01$) for those candidates who chose to use a Baha as a CROS device permanently.

Bone-anchored hearing aids (Baha) have been used for over 30 years for the treatment of conductive or mixed hearing losses [1, 2] and for some 10 years for the treatment of single-sided sensorineural deafness (SSD) by means of transcranial contralateral routing of signals or CROS [3, 4]. The Baha titanium implant, which is placed retroauricularly, allows reliable and efficient sound transmission to the contralateral inner ear.

The benefit of transcranial CROS fittings in patients with SSD has been reported by a number of studies [5–7]. The main effect is to reduce acoustic head shadow and to provide better signal-to-noise ratios, depending on the spatial distribution of the signal and noise sources. Outcomes in Baha CROS fittings have been reported to be superior to conventional CROS fittings [4].

Despite the proven benefits and its general success, it has been estimated for some etiologies that <20% of the patients would choose a Baha CROS if given the opportunity [8]. To date, we cannot predict with reasonable certainty which candidates will choose a Baha CROS and which will decline. In patients with unilateral conductive deafness, it has been shown that the benefit tends to be smaller for patients with a longstanding hearing loss than for those with a more recently acquired hearing loss [9]. For SSD, the work by Martin et al. [10] suggests, in contrast, that users with a congenital hearing loss benefit more from a Baha. Stenfelt [11] suggested that the benefit of a Baha CROS should be greater for users with smaller transcranial attenuations.

In this study, we analyzed the preoperative data of 46 Baha CROS candidates and correlated their age, etiology and duration of deafness, hearing thresholds and transcranial attenuation with their decision for or against a permanent Baha CROS fitting after a trial-at-home period. In addition, a new questionnaire, the Bern Benefit in Single-Sided Deafness (BBSS) is presented, and the correlation of the answers of 28 candidates with their decision for or against a Baha is investigated.

Materials and Methods

The data of 46 patients (mean age 48.4 years, range 18.8–78.9) who were counseled at our department between 2004 and 2010 for a Baha CROS were analyzed. All candidates had a considerable sensorineural hearing loss in one ear (25 right, 21 left) and a normal or almost normal hearing in the other hear. Candidates who were referred to our center explicitly for a Baha CROS evaluation but were borderline cases on the basis of their audiograms were included as far as possible, resulting in a relatively broad range of hearing thresholds, as will be shown later in the chapter.

All candidates had the possibility to test a Baha with a headband in their normal environment for a 7- to 10-day trial period. At the end of this trial, 17 of the 46 candidates declined further use of a Baha, and 29 patients decided to have a Baha system implanted and became permanent users. Four patients were fitted with a Baha® Compact [12], 3 with a Baha® Intenso [13], and 22 with a Baha® Divino [12] sound processor.

Pure tone hearing thresholds were measured in all subjects. On the basis of the suggestion by Stenfelt [11], the transcranial attenuation was measured in a subset of 38 candidates. The unmasked bone conduction thresholds were measured at 250, 500, 1,000, 2,000, 3,000, and 4,000 Hz, and the values obtained with the bone vibrator placed either behind the poorer or behind the better ears were subtracted.

Table 1. Age and sex of the study population

	Baha chosen (n = 29)	Baha declined (n = 17)
Age, years	50.2 (18.8–78.9)	45.4 (24.4–63.2)
Male	17	10
Female	12	7

Values for age are expressed as mean (range).

To help the candidates assess the benefit of the Baha during the trial-at-home period, we developed the BBSS questionnaire consisting of 10 visual analogue scales. The idea behind the BBSS was to help candidates for a conventional or Baha CROS hearing aid consciously rate the benefit of their device in several different and relevant environments. The BBSS was administered in 28 patients. The questionnaire is currently available in English, German, French, Italian, Slovak and Arabic, and can be downloaded at www.hno.insel.ch/BBSS.html. The English version can be found in the appendix.

All audiometric measurements took place in a sound-proof chamber (Type 402A; industrial Acoustics Company, Niederkrüchten, Germany) using a GSI 61 audiometer (Grason-Stadler, Milford, N.H., USA) and a type B-71 (Radioear, New Eagle, Pa., USA) bone vibrator. Data were analyzed by a certified statistician (M.K.) using the Instat 3.10 software package (GraphPad Inc, San Diego, Calif., USA).

Results

Table 1 shows the relation between age, sex and the decision for or against a Baha CROS system. Candidates who chose a Baha were slightly older ($p = 0.28$, unpaired two-sided Mann-Whitney test). No difference was found between the decisions of men and women (Fisher's exact test, two-tailed $p = 1.0$).

Table 2 shows the etiologies for the SSD. Again, no specific differences between candidates who chose or who declined a Baha were found.

Figure 1 shows the distribution of the duration of deafness. The distribution was similar for both

Table 2. Etiology of sudden hearing loss and decision

	Baha chosen	Baha declined	Total
Sudden hearing loss	8	6	14
Unknown, congenital	5	4	9
Unknown, later onset	4	0	4
Infection[1]	3	3	6
Trauma	4	1	5
Acoustic neuroma	2	2	4
Post-ear surgery	3	0	3
Otosclerosis	0	1	1
Total	29	17	46

[1]Three mumps, 1 herpes zoster oticus, 2 unspecified otitis, with no further information available.

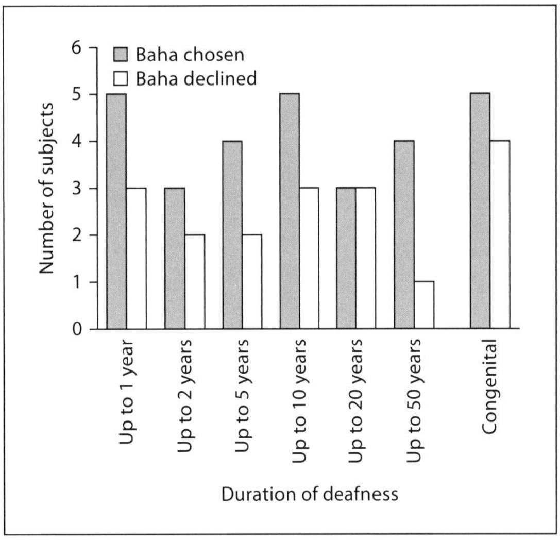

Fig. 1. Distribution of the duration of deafness for the subgroups who chose and declined a Baha.

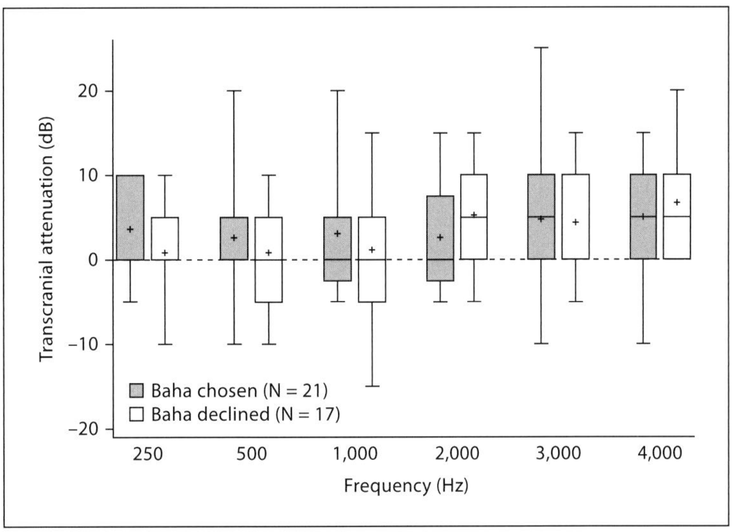

Fig. 2. Distribution of the transcranial attenuation in the two study groups. Data are shown as quartiles (boxes), medians (horizontal lines in boxes), mean values (+), minima and maxima.

groups of patients. The average duration of deafness was 16.0 years for those who wanted a Baha and 15.5 years for those who decided against it. The difference was not statistically significant (unpaired two-sided Mann-Whitney test $p = 0.97$).

Figure 2 shows the distribution of the transcranial attenuation of 38 candidates. There was a wide spread between –15 and +25 dB. Attenuations tended to be more pronounced at higher frequencies (average of 5.79 dB at 4,000

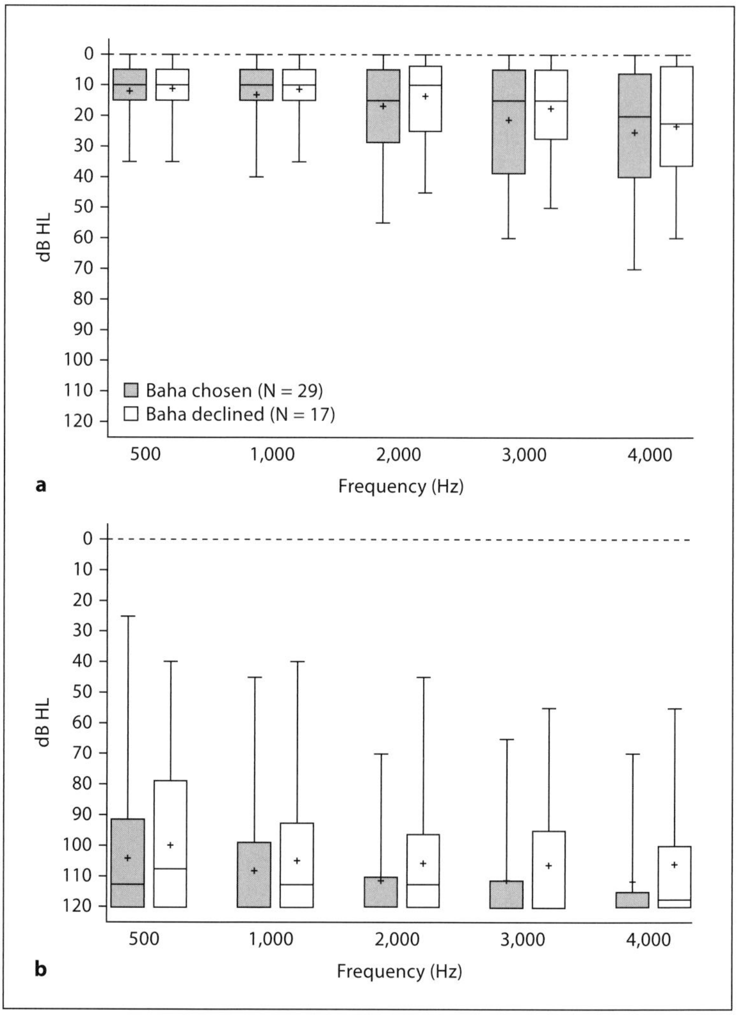

Fig. 3. Air conduction hearing thresholds in better (**a**) and poorer (**b**) ears. Data are shown as quartiles (boxes), medians (horizontal lines in boxes), mean values (+), minima and maxima. None of the differences between those candidates who chose and those who declined Baha are statistically significant. Extreme values show measurements from different candidates at different frequencies and do not represent the threshold of any single subject.

Hz) and smaller at lower frequencies (average of 1.67 dB at 500 Hz).

Transcranial attenuations were similar in both groups. In 4 out of the 6 frequencies tested, average attenuations were slightly smaller for the subjects who subsequently declined a Baha. However, the difference was not statistically significant at any frequency (unpaired two-sided Mann-Whitney test, p = 0.19–0.87)

Figure 3 shows the distribution of the air conduction thresholds of both groups. The hearing thresholds of the better ear were similar in those who subsequently chose to use a Baha permanently and those who declined it. Thresholds in the poorer ear were a little better for the subjects who declined a Baha CROS, especially at frequencies above 2,000 Hz. Nevertheless, none of the differences was statistically significant (unpaired two-sided Mann-Whitney test, p = 0.30–0.97).

Two of the candidates who were given the BBSS questionnaire did not return it. Both reported testing the device only in a few situations,

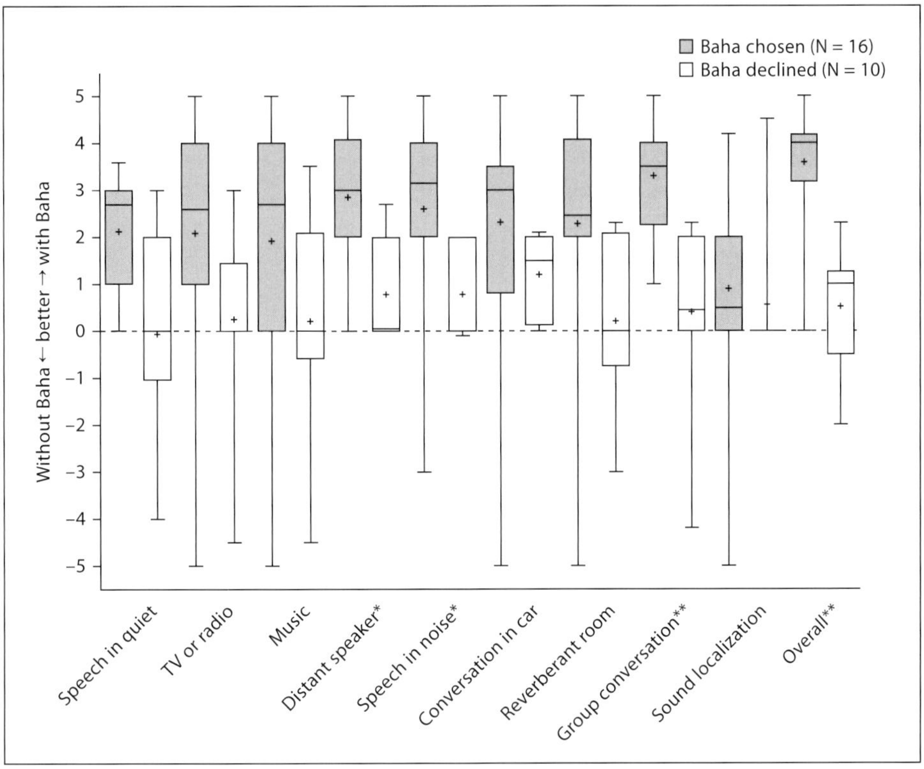

Fig. 4. Distribution of the answers to the BBSS questionnaire. Data are shown as quartiles (boxes), medians (horizontal lines in boxes), mean values (+), minima and maxima. Asterisks denote statistically significant differences (*p < 0.05, **p < 0.01).

and both decided against a Baha. Figure 4 shows a synopsis of the answers of the remaining 26 subjects who received a BBSS questionnaire.

In all 10 questions, hearing with a Baha was rated more positively on average by the candidates who subsequently chose a Baha than by those who declined it. The difference was statistically significant for 4 of the 10 questions: speaker at a distance (difference +2.0 points, p = 0.026), speech in noise (+1.8 points, p = 0.037), group conversation (+2.9 points, p = 0.002) and overall assessment (+3.1 points, p = 0.002, unpaired two-sided Mann-Whitney test with Bonferroni correction). The smallest average difference of +0.3 points was reported for sound localization (p = 0.16).

When the scores of all 10 questions were added, the total score ranged from +5.5 to +41.0 (mean: 25.1, standard deviation 10.2) for those in favor of a Baha, and –18.2 to +15.8 (mean: 4.4, standard deviation 9.7) for those who declined a Baha. The difference was statistically highly significant (p = 0.0003, unpaired two-sided Mann-Whitney test).

Discussion

In our group of candidates, we found no evidence that age, sex, the etiology or duration of the deafness, transcranial attenuation, or hearing thresholds had any significant influence on the decision for or against a permanent Baha CROS fitting. Hearing threshold also had no statistical significance. Specifically, a long-standing or even a congenital hearing loss does not seem to affect the decision for a Baha CROS negatively. This is in line with the findings by Martin et al. [10].

Transcranial attenuations increased for higher frequencies, as expected [14]. Despite substantial differences between individuals, there is no evidence that this is a predictive factor regarding the decision for or against Baha CROS. Contrary to expectation [11], on average, candidates who chose a Baha even had (slightly and non-significantly) lower transcranial attenuations.

The BBSS questionnaire was developed to help patients assess CROS hearing aids. In addition, we found that the answers can predict the decision for or against a Baha in SSD. Of all the parameters considered in this study, the data from the BBSS show the highest correlation with the subsequent decision. The fact that the Baha is assessed more positively by those who chose a Baha on all 10 scales suggests that a generally positive attitude towards the device may have influenced all answers. On average, the smallest benefit was reported for sound localization. This is in line with several reports showing no improvement in sound localization due to Baha CROS [5]. The largest differences between those who chose a Baha and those who declined it can be found for speech understanding in situations where competing acoustic signals are present or likely to be present.

A decision for or against a Baha system involves more than just the weighing of hearing benefits. Additional aspects, such as the implantation of the titanium implant or cosmetic considerations are not covered by the questionnaire. However, if the answers to all 10 questions are added, the total score gives an idea of the relative weighting. Total scores of 15 or higher seem to indicate situations where the perceived hearing benefit is likely to outweigh possible issues with regard to Baha. For values below 10, most candidates decide against the use of a Baha.

Appendix

The BBSS Questionnaire

Please rate your perceived benefit from your aid in the following situations by a vertical line. Example:

Much easier without the aid			... somewhat easier		Similar with and without		... somewhat easier		Much easier with the aid	
–5	–4	–3	–2	–1	0	1	2	3	4	5

1. To hold a conversation with one person in a quiet environment. For me, this is:

Much easier without the aid			... somewhat easier		Similar with and without		... somewhat easier		Much easier with the aid	
–5	–4	–3	–2	–1	0	1	2	3	4	5

2. To understand a TV or a radio speaker. For me, this is:

Much easier without the aid	... somewhat easier	Similar with and without	... somewhat easier	Much easier with the aid

–5 –4 –3 –2 –1 0 1 2 3 4 5

3. To listen to music. For me, this is:

Much more pleasant without the aid	... somewhat more pleasant	Similar with and without	... somewhat more pleasant	Much more pleasant with the aid

–5 –4 –3 –2 –1 0 1 2 3 4 5

4. To follow a conversation from some distance (5 m/15 ft or more). For me, this is:

Much easier without the aid	... somewhat easier	Similar with and without	... somewhat easier	Much easier with the aid

–5 –4 –3 –2 –1 0 1 2 3 4 5

5. To follow a conversation with background noise. For me, this is:

Much easier without the aid	... somewhat easier	Similar with and without	... somewhat easier	Much easier with the aid

–5 –4 –3 –2 –1 0 1 2 3 4 5

6. To hold a conversation while driving in a car. For me, this is:

Much easier without the aid	... somewhat easier	Similar with and without	... somewhat easier	Much easier with the aid

–5 –4 –3 –2 –1 0 1 2 3 4 5

7. To understand speech in a reverberant room, such as a large entrance hall or a church. For me, this is:

Much easier without the aid	... somewhat easier	Similar with and without	... somewhat easier	Much easier with the aid

–5 –4 –3 –2 –1 0 1 2 3 4 5

8. To participate in a group conversation with 3 or more participants. For me, this is:

Much easier without the aid			... somewhat easier		Similar with and without		... somewhat easier		Much easier with the aid	
–5	–4	–3	–2	–1	0	1	2	3	4	5

9. To localize a sound source, such as a honking car. For me, this is:

Much easier without the aid			... somewhat easier		Similar with and without		... somewhat easier		Much easier with the aid	
–5	–4	–3	–2	–1	0	1	2	3	4	5

10. Overall, for me hearing is:

Much better without the aid			... somewhat better		Similar with and without		... somewhat better		Much better with the aid	
–5	–4	–3	–2	–1	0	1	2	3	4	5

Acknowledgements

We would like to thank Prof. Dr. D. Koval, Prof. Dr. D. Vibert, Dr. H. Aloraibi, and Ms. E. Tundo for their translations of the BBSS questionnaire and Ms. E. Clamann for her translation of the English version and proofreading the manuscript.

References

1 Tjellström A, Rosenhall U, Lindström J, Hallén O, Albrektsson T, Brånemark PI: Five-year experience with skin-penetrating bone-anchored implants in the temporal bone. Acta Otolaryngol 1983;95:568–575.

2 Håkansson B, Lidén G, Tjellström A, Ringdahl A, Jacobsson M, Carlsson P, Erlandson BE: Ten years of experience with the Swedish bone-anchored hearing system. Ann Otol Rhinol Laryngol Suppl 1990;151:1–16.

3 Niparko JK, Cox KM, Lustig LR: Comparison of the bone anchored hearing aid implantable hearing device with contralateral routing of offside signal amplification in the rehabilitation of unilateral deafness. Otol Neurotol 2003;24:73–78.

4 Wazen JJ, Spitzer JB, Ghossaini SN, Fayad JN, Niparko JK, Cox K, Brackmann DE, Soli SD: Transcranial contralateral cochlear stimulation in unilateral deafness. Otolaryngol Head Neck Surg 2003;129:248–254.

5 Hol MK, Bosman AJ, Snik AF, Mylanus EA, Cremers CW: Bone-anchored hearing aid in unilateral inner ear deafness: a study of 20 patients. Audiol Neurootol 2004;9:274–281.

6 Pfiffner F, Kompis M, Stieger C: Bone-anchored hearing aids: correlation between pure-tone thresholds and outcome in three user groups. Otol Neurotol 2009;30:884–890.

7 Wazen JJ, Van Ess MJ, Alameda J, Ortega C, Modisett M, Pinsky K: The Baha system in patients with single sided deafness and contralateral hearing loss. Otolarngol Head Neck Surg 2010;142:554–559.

8 Schrøder SA, Ravn T, Bonding P: BAHA in single-sided deafness: patient compliance and subjective benefit. Otol Neurotol 2010;31:404–408.

9 Snik AF, Mylanus EA, Cremers CW: The bone-anchored hearing aid in patients with a unilateral air-bone gap. Otol Neurotol 2002;23:61–66.

10 Martin TP, Lowther R, Cooper H, Holder RL, Irving RM, Reid AP, Proops DW: The bone-anchored hearing aid in the rehabilitation of single-sided deafness: experience with 58 patients. Clin Otolaryngol 2010;35:284–290.
11 Stenfelt S: Bilateral fitting of BAHAs and BAHA fitted in unilateral deaf persons: acoustical aspects. Int J Audiol 2005;44:178–189.
12 Kompis M, Krebs M, Häusler R: Speech understanding in quiet and in noise with the bone-anchored hearing aids Baha Compact and Baha Divino. Acta Otolaryngol 2007;127:829–835.
13 Bosman AJ, Snik FM, Mylanus EA, Cremers WR: Fitting range of the BAHA Intenso. Int J Audiol 2009;48:346–352.
14 Nolan M, Lyon DJ: Transcranial attenuation in bone conduction audiometry. J Laryngol Otol 1981;95:597–608.

Prof. Martin Kompis, MD, PhD
Department of ENT, Head and Neck Surgery, Inselspital, University of Bern
CH–3010 Bern (Switzerland)
Tel. +41 31 632 33 00, Fax +41 31 632 31 93, E-Mail martin.kompis@insel.ch

Kompis M, Caversaccio M-D (eds): Implantable Bone Conduction Hearing Aids.
Adv Otorhinolaryngol. Basel, Karger, 2011, vol 71, pp 112–123

Challenges and Recent Developments in Sound Processing for Baha®

Mark C. Flynn

Cochlear Bone Anchored Solutions AB, Göteborg, Sweden

Abstract

Osseointegrated auditory implants such as Baha® provide an efficient pathway for sound delivery and an excellent amplification choice for patients with conductive or mixed hearing loss or single-sided sensorineural deafness. But at the same time, bone conduction hearing provides a number of key challenges that need to be addressed. One solution is computer-based fitting software to measure in-situ thresholds directly through the Baha sound processor and to individually prescribe amplification settings based on the patient's hearing loss and degree of transcranial attenuation. Additionally, technologies such as automatic directional microphones and noise reduction systems further improve hearing performance in noisy situations. This paper highlights recent technological innovations and summarizes data on the advantages for the Baha patient population using the sound processing capabilities available in the latest Baha sound processors.

Baha® offers a comprehensive hearing solution for adults and children with conductive or mixed hearing loss or single-sided sensorineural deafness (SSD). The Baha system consists of a sound processor, osseointegrated titanium implant and an abutment connecting the system as described in the chapter by Stewart et al. [this vol.]. Each aspect of the system has been the result of systematic investigation. For example, in terms of the implant, recent clinical (n = 77) [1] and preclinical (n = 60) [2, 3] data were published on the new Baha 3 system implant (Cochlear™ Baha BI300). These reports conclude that the new implant is (a) significantly more stable, and (b) has faster osseointegration than the previous Branemark implant at any time period. Improvements in implant technology such as the TioBlast™ surface, small-sized threads and increased diameter provide important benefits to the patient.

Similarly, new Baha sound processors have become available that offer many new technical and audiological applications designed to meet the needs of the hearing-impaired person. Earlier speech processors developed for Baha were, for the most part, relatively straightforward single-channel hearing devices, with little additional functionality. The latest generation of sound processors (e.g. Cochlear Baha BP100) offers multiple channels of acoustic sound processing, advanced signal processing technology (i.e. automatic directional microphones and noise reduction circuits) and the capability for fitting using computer-based software. Recently, there have been positive reports of improved speech recognition and perceived sound quality for patients wearing Baha using these new sound processing schemes [4–7].

In order to systematically evaluate the sound processor capabilities and technology building blocks, a conceptual framework must be presented. There are three aspects of Baha sound processing that will be evaluated in this paper. First, an examination of pre-processing features that clean the signal for later amplification in the processor. Second, how that signal is processed and amplified, including what tools the hearing care professional has to further individualize the processor for the patient. Third, how bone conduction provides a number of advantages over air conduction hearing for people with conductive and mixed hearing loss and SSD.

Cleaning the Signal

Prior to compensating for the hearing loss, the incoming signal can be pre-processed, so that the best possible signal is available for amplification. This pre-processing could be seen as analogous to a cleaning of the signal. Patients with Baha require three aspects of sound cleaning. First, adjustments should be made for the position relative to the pinna as the Baha is worn posterior to the auricle. Second, directional microphone technology can be used to improve the signal-to-noise ratio (SNR). Third, automatic noise reduction technology is implemented to ensure that noise does not distract the listener.

Position Compensation

The Baha sound processor is worn 5–6 cm posterior to the ear canal, and the actual microphone is angled towards the back of the head with sound from the front being acoustically shielded by the pinna. Therefore, the listener's soundscape is compromised, as sounds from the front and rear are not weighted equally. Therefore, sounds from the rear will be more audible than sounds from in front [8]. This provides the strange sensation of having improved speech understanding (in the absence of visual cues) and audibility when speech is from the back rather than in front of the listener.

Given the advances in signal processing and the use of two microphones, the time delay can be adjusted to compensate for the postauricular Baha position. In essence, a slight directionality is created to provide the listener with a true omnidirectional signal when worn on the abutment. As sounds are equalized from around the listener, the result will be that sounds are now calibrated in loudness from all directions to mimic the directivity of natural hearing.

A direct measure of improvement was demonstrated by Flynn [9] who investigated the use of this feature with speech presented from the front loudspeaker and noise from the rear loudspeaker. Using the adaptive HINT (Hearing In Noise Test) [10] procedure, significant improvement in speech understanding in noise with the position compensation turned on versus off was demonstrated [$F(1, 21) = 6.95$, $p < 0.05$]. Similarly, interpretation of the data presented by Kompis and Pfiffner [6] reported the benefits of the position compensation for 20 adults using the Cochlear Baha BP100 Sound Processor compared with Cochlear Divino™ (Cochlear Bone Anchored Solutions AB, Sweden). Importantly, the authors confirmed that the use of technology, such as position compensation, did not compromise directional microphone performance, as the same degree of directional microphone benefit was measured with BP100 and Divino. As position compensation can be disabled (e.g. advised if the BP100 is worn on a Softband on the frontal bone), measurement of benefit is easy to determine in a speech in noise test. Position compensation adjusts for the position of the Baha on the head, thereby equalizing the relative intensity of sounds from the front and back to offer an improved soundscape and speech understanding in the omnidirectional microphone mode.

Directional Microphones

Directional microphones are the only sound-processing technology shown to enhance the SNR for hearing-impaired individuals [11–14]. The underlying principle for any directional microphone system is based on the necessity for the noise and signal to be spatially separated. The assumption is made that the important signal (i.e. speech) is from the frontal cardiod directivity pattern, while noise is from the back cardiod of the listener and can therefore be attenuated.

Directional microphones have been available for Baha as either an additional connection (for the early model Baha Classic sound processor) or built in (Cochlear Baha BP100 or Baha Divino). A number of studies have measured the benefits of the directional microphone for Baha. Blackmore et al. [15] reported data from 11 patients who wore the directional microphone as a plug-in accessory. They found that the directional microphone led to a significant improvement in the overall quality of life as measured on the Glasgow Benefit Inventory. At the same time, Kompis et al. [11] evaluated hearing performance in 7 Baha Divino users who had bilateral substantial conductive or mixed hearing losses. Performance was measured using an adaptive sentence test in noise (Basler sentence test) to determine the SNR for 50% speech recognition. They found, on average, a 1.9-dB improvement in SNR when speech was presented from the front (0°) and noise from behind (180°). Kompis et al. [11] noted that while subjects demonstrated benefit in the test situation, not all subjects reported using the directional microphone in their daily life because the requirement to manually switch to the directional microphone program was considered too cumbersome.

Thus far, studies have focused on patients with conductive or mixed hearing loss; this raises the important question of whether patients with SSD also benefit from a directional microphone. To address this, Oeding et al. [16] measured the performance of 16 SSD patients using Baha with and without the directional microphone. Performance was measured with speech from the front and when noise was at 180° behind the listener or for an eight-loudspeaker array (45° separation between the speech and noise), and with the good ear both open and closed using a hearing protector muff. The authors reported an average 2.6-dB improvement in the SNR for 50% speech recognition in noise with activation of the directional microphone. The benefit was observed with the good ear either open or closed, and with either the diffuse or single-speaker test set-up. Therefore, the use of a directional microphone provides significant benefit for patients wearing Baha, irrespective of the indication. One common concern, however, is that a number of patients report that they find manual switching to be too bothersome to use in everyday life [11, 17].

To address this concern, recent Baha sound processors implement a directional system that is both automatic and adaptive [18–21] (fig. 1). *Automatic* refers to the ability to automatically switch between the omnidirectional and directional microphone settings (as opposed to manual systems where the listener presses a button). *Adaptive* refers to the shape of the polar plot when the device is in a directional mode. The microphone polar plots are continuously updated to provide the greatest reduction in noise. The ability of the polar pattern to adapt to the unique configuration of each sound environment provides improved performance over systems where the polar response remains fixed to a certain predetermined pattern [18–24]. In one implementation, as processing occurs in the time domain, the polar response is varied by frequency so that multiple noise sources are attenuated simultaneously.

For this more advanced directional microphone system, an initial report by Flynn et al. [4] detailed an average SNR improvement of 2.4 dB for 50% speech recognition of sentence materials using a

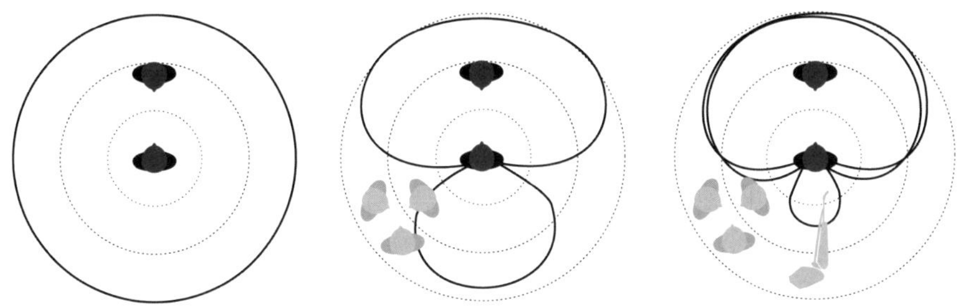

Fig. 1. Illustration of omnidirectional, single-band fixed directional and multiple-band adaptive directional microphone possibilities. The number of bands adapts to the number of distinct noise sources detected in the sound environment.

Swedish version of the HINT test [10]. Similarly, a study performed by Kompis and Pfiffner [6] on 20 patients with conductive or mixed hearing loss reported a similar average SNR improvement of 2.3 dB. Importantly, the relative differences between omnidirectional and directional microphone settings for Divino and BP100 were identical. Using the estimation provided by Dillon [25], where each 1 dB improvement in signal-to-noise ratio provides a 10% improvement in speech understanding. Therefore, the directional microphone provides a clinically relevant >20% improvement in speech understanding in noise.

Noise Management Circuits

When the noise is very loud (i.e. poor SNR) and/or coming from the same direction as the speech, a directional microphone may not provide improved speech recognition. To reduce the annoyance of such high-level noisy environments, the latest Baha sound processors analyze the degree of modulation and input sound level in each channel. Speech has a high degree of modulation compared to noise, so the assumption is that any channel with a low degree of modulation contains little or no speech information. Thus, the effect of noise in that channel can be reduced, for example by reducing gain or through spectral subtraction. To preserve the intelligibility of speech, the amount of reduction in a channel is tempered by the Speech Intelligibility Index. While modulation detection circuitry can accurately detect a noise-dominated channel, reports in the research literature discuss that this type of algorithm has limitations in separating noise from speech [26–28]. Therefore, the purpose is to reduce the impact of noise rather than to improve intelligibility per se [28].

However, there does exist a possibility for a specific setting for patients with SSD to actually improve speech understanding. For patients with SSD, when the noise arrives principally at the ear with the Baha, the Baha may inadvertently amplify the noise so that it masks a signal with a better SNR that arrives at the good ear. Noise reduction circuits can provide a solution in this scenario. When a signal with high intensity level and low modulation is received by the Baha, a more aggressive noise reduction strategy can be applied. For SSD, the degree of noise reduction is increased to ensure that the Baha does not significantly worsen the SNR at the functioning cochlea when noise is to the Baha ear and speech to the good ear. This application may lessen the masking effect of listening situations where noise is to the Baha side and speech to the good side [29–32].

Automatic Feedback Cancellation
Avoiding feedback is an important consideration in the design and development of Baha sound processors. Acoustic and mechanical feedback limits the overall gain of the Baha sound processor. As the sound processor approaches the threshold of feedback, a ringing or metallic sound quality will be produced. The sound processor will start to oscillate (howl) if the gain is increased beyond this limit. In the past, the only solution was to reduce or limit the gain either by limiting the overall gain or by instructing the patient to turn down the volume.

Unlike hearing aids where feedback is typically restricted to approximately 2,000–5,000 Hz [33], the feedback challenge in Baha comes from at least four sources which vary in nature and across the frequency spectrum. First, there is acoustic feedback in the high frequencies. Second, mechanical feedback originates from the transducer which is typically lower in frequency. Third, feedback related to shifting of the resonance peak of the transducer when, for example, the Baha sound processor is worn on a Softband versus an abutment. Fourth, the feedback path is altered by the distance of the Baha sound processor from the soft tissue and pinna.

These challenges make Baha dedicated feedback cancellation solutions a necessity in modern Baha design. Similar to Cochlear Baha Intenso^{TM}, Cochlear Baha BP100 uses active feedback cancellation (AFC) to increase the feedback margin for mechanical and acoustical feedback. Briefly, AFC allows for rapid identification and elimination of feedback without a noticeable degradation in sound quality. Whenever feedback occurs, it is immediately detected. The feedback 'howl' is then reduced through phase cancellation. Importantly, unlike hearing aid applications, the AFC has a broad bandwidth and is applied across multiple channels due to the sources of feedback discussed previously. This feedback reduction system also detects and limits the amplification for different frequencies so that the gain for each individual frequency band stays below the limits of controllable gain within the feedback cancellation system. This provides additional gain at important frequencies which should then provide the patient with increased audibility and less occurrences of feedback compared to previous generations of Baha sound processors for the same fitting range.

Dedicated Amplification for Bone Conduction

The very nature of bone conduction necessitates that we develop hearing solutions designed specifically for amplification of sound through bone. In many cases, such as a person with a pure conductive hearing loss or normal hearing in the contralateral ear with SSD, we build hearing solutions for patients who have a normal cochlea. Even for severe mixed hearing loss, where the air conduction threshold may be around 90 dB HL, the bone conduction hearing loss is <65 dB HL, and in most cases can be around 30–50 dB HL. As Baha will send the signal directly to the cochlea and bypass any outer and middle ear pathology, the degree of hearing loss to be compensated is relatively mild compared with typical hearing aid users.

Fitting Baha Sound Processors
The approach of prescribing required gain based on the patient's bone conduction thresholds is a recent innovation for Baha. Previously, Baha sound processors were essentially fitted to most

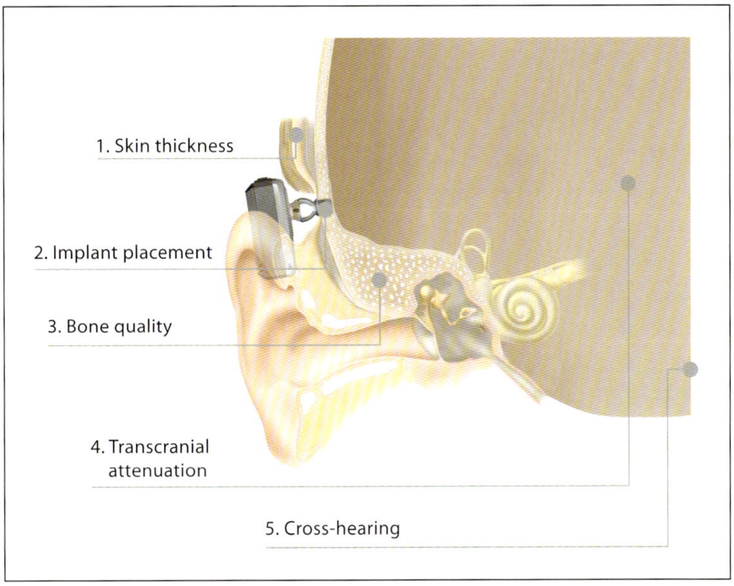

Fig. 2. Sources of the five areas of audiometric variability in a Baha fitting.

comfortable listening level using inbuilt trimpots. Today, Baha sound processors are fitted via computer-based fitting software. This aligns Baha sound processors with other auditory hearing devices, such as hearing aids, middle ear implants and cochlear implants that use fitting software. To simplify fitting, the twelve sound processing channels are mapped to the ten audiometric frequencies (250, 500, 750, 1,000, 1,500, 2,000, 3,000, 4,000, 6,000, and 8,000 Hz). For each channel, soft gain (40 dB SPL input), loud gain (60 dB SPL input) and maximum power output can be adjusted individually to allow more accurate fitting than is available with the adjustment of a low cut and gain trimmer in previous devices. In addition, the fitting software allows a greater scope for individualizing the sound processor to meet each patient's needs, such as through multiple user-selectable listening programs (e.g. typically 'music', 'noise', and 'everyday' settings), configuration of how the sound processor should treat external sound inputs (e.g. iPod™, cell phone, FM systems) and configuration of settings related to beeps (frequency and loudness), visual indicators, and tamper-resistant controls.

Measurement of Bone Conduction Thresholds Directly through the Sound Processor

It is important to fit bone conduction sound processors based on the patient's direct thresholds (i.e. through abutment or band) rather than indirect thresholds (interpretation from audiogram). This ensures than any uncontrolled variability is removed. In Baha fittings, variability arises from potentially five factors, as illustrated in figure 2. First, the thickness of the skin impacts the efficiency of transmission [34]. Second, the placement of the bone transducer or Baha implant may vary between patients, affecting the distance to the cochlea [35]. Third, transmission of sound may be affected by bone quality and thickness. Fourth, as noted previously, there is a large degree of individual variability in terms of transcranial attenuation (TCA) [36]. Fifth, the amount of cross-hearing will vary depending on hearing levels in the contralateral cochlea.

To overcome this variability, a Baha sound processor should be designed to allow the measurement of bone conduction thresholds directly. This reduces the variability caused by the factors discussed above. The Cochlear Baha Fitting Software allows the accurate collection of direct BC thresholds as part of the fitting process using a software feature called BC Direct. Pure-tone signals at different intensities (dB HL) and frequencies (Hz) are presented through the sound processor. The test measurement techniques are similar to those used for a standard audiogram. Therefore, the patient's actual bone conduction thresholds are measured so that the amount of variability is reduced and prescription-based fittings are more accurate.

In sum, sound processor measurement of direct bone conduction thresholds (e.g. BC Direct) offers three advantages over traditional bone conduction audiometry. First, it eliminates the variability of stimulator placement and skin thickness by transmitting the test tone directly through the implant. Second, it eliminates the need for masking, as the purpose is to determine the softest sounds audible through the Baha sound processor. Third, no extra equipment is required other than the BP100 sound processor and Cochlear Baha Fitting Software on a stand alone or portable computer. In most instances, the four most important test frequencies (500, 1,000, 2,000 and 4,000 Hz) can be measured quickly and simply in only a few minutes. Given the ambiguity of converting between indirect and direct measurements of bone transmission, measurement of direct bone conduction thresholds are recommended for all Baha fittings.

Adapting Multiple Channel Nonlinear Amplification for Baha

Multiple-channel nonlinear amplification refers to two distinct sound processing advantages over the single-channel linear processing found in previous generations of Baha sound processors. First, nonlinear amplification provides a more sensible [25] method of amplification through applying gain differentially depending on the input sound level and the user's needs. Typically, nonlinear amplification compresses the output signal so that soft sounds (e.g. consonants) receive a relative increase in gain, whereas louder sounds (e.g. traffic noise) receive less gain. This avoids the situation in the previous linear approach whereby all sounds receive exactly the same amplification. Overall, this approach compresses the input sound into the user's residual dynamic range and provides better speech understanding in noise and overall audibility [25, 37, 39].

Second, the earlier generations of Baha sound processors (e.g. Baha Divino and Intenso), were single-channel devices. Thereby, a change in sound level at one frequency affects the gain in all other frequencies. For example, a loud sound at one frequency (e.g. low-frequency traffic noise) will effect the amplification at other frequencies (e.g. high-frequency consonants), distorting the sound scene and potentially reducing intelligibility. By dividing the input signal into a number of discrete channels, gain can be applied judiciously so that changes in level in one frequency region do not interfere with the required amplification at other frequencies. Similarly, the gain can be specifically prescribed or adjusted so that the amplification is matched to the slope of the hearing loss or the patient's unique bone conduction characteristics.

Combined together, research reports conclude that the combination of multiple-channel nonlinear amplification provides significant hearing performance benefits for adults [38–42] and children [43, 44].

Requirement of a High Maximum Power Output

A known limitation of Baha is the amount of amplification that can be provided to the patient before the maximum output is reached. This was a critical issue in older Baha sound processor designs. Although it may be argued that maximum output should be higher, in a hearing aid the output limiting is typically designed to be reached at

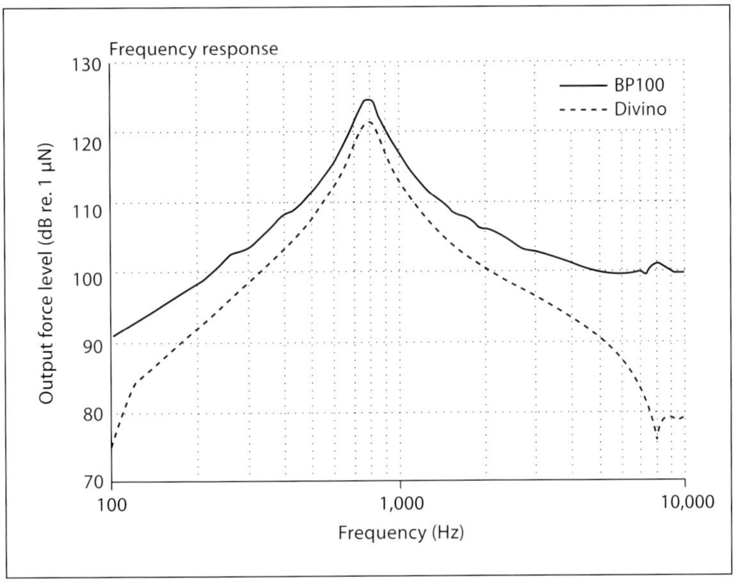

Fig. 3. Comparison of the maximum power output between the Baha Divino and the Cochlear Baha BP100. Figure printed with permission from Cochlear Bone Anchored Solutions AB, Sweden.

approximately 90 dB SPL (i.e. OSPL 90). For Baha, however, the sound processor has often reached the output limits at relatively low input level – occasionally around 70 dB SPL at the higher frequencies. This situation creates difficulties for the hearing-impaired person in challenging listening situations. If the output does not change with input, then the benefit of any positive signal-to-noise level is lost and the loudness growth is limited. It is therefore imperative to develop transducers with greater output power. To this end, a new transducer was developed for Cochlear Baha BP100 to provide significantly greater output power than any other Baha sound processor designed for the same fitting range (up to and including 45 dB HL; fig. 3 and 4). In conclusion, required amplification will no longer be limited by output compression in most communication situations.

Dedicated Hearing Loss Prescription for Baha
Hearing losses vary in terms of degree, configuration and type. Therefore, amplification requirements need to be adjusted to fit the individual patient's hearing loss. There is no single setting that

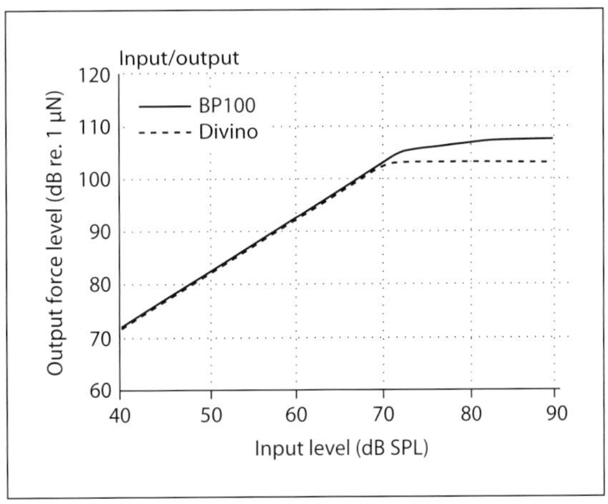

Fig. 4. Comparison of input/output curves at 1,600 Hz between the Baha Divino and the Cochlear Baha BP100 (for comparison, both devices in linear test mode and full on gain). The importance of increased maximum power output is clearly shown here as BP100 has significantly greater headroom and does not introduce output compression as early. Figure printed with permission from Cochlear Bone Anchored Solutions AB, Sweden.

is good for all patients. A prescriptive approach offers the only practical method for determining the optimum settings [25]. In short, the prescriptive approach takes in the known characteristics of the patient's hearing loss and determines, based on empirical evidence, the degree of compensation required.

For air conduction, it is generally assumed that the amount of gain required to compensate for hearing loss is approximately half the threshold loss [45]. This requirement is challenged for bone conduction devices where the loudness growth is 10–20% greater through bone conduction than air conduction [46]. Therefore, the amount of gain required for any given cochlea loss is less for bone conduction than air conduction. Based on this requirement, hearing aid amplifications strategies such as NAL-NL1 and DSL v5.0 would clearly be inappropriate for direct bone conduction as they would overamplify sound for the patient. This is hardly surprising as conventional hearing aids are designed for an intact pathway with an impaired cochlea. The Baha is designed for an impaired pathway with, for the most part, an intact cochlea.

Therefore, direct bone conduction requires an amplification strategy such as the Cochlear Baha Prescription which takes into account the loudness growth of bone conduction. The BP100 implements this prescription across twelve channels using a multiple-channel nonlinear approach. Gain is applied differently depending on the input sound level and the user's needs. For a hearing impaired person, the dynamic range becomes compressed, so that there is a more limited dynamic range than expected. Nonlinear amplification thereby compresses the output signal so that soft sounds (e.g. consonants) receive a relative increase in gain, whereas louder sounds (e.g. traffic noise) receive relatively less gain. Overall, this approach compresses the input sound into the user's residual dynamic range and provides better speech understanding in noise and overall audibility [25, 37, 38].

For SSD, the assumptions discussed above regarding applicability and required amplification remain the same. An important consideration, however, is that the skull attenuates sound as it is transferred from the Baha side to the good hearing cochlea on the contralateral side [36, 47]. This effect is labeled transcranial attenuation (TCA). The effect results in current Baha wearers using a louder volume control setting than would be estimated from the thresholds in the better hearing ear. To ease fitting, the average values such as those from Nolan and Lyon [36] are added directly to the prescribed gain, so that the desired amount of compensation is achieved. If direct bone conduction thresholds are available, then the patient's actual (rather than estimated) TCA values are used.

This means that difficulties experienced with SSD are principally a result of the head shadow effect, where the high-frequency sounds are attenuated by up to 20 dB SPL and the low-frequency sounds are not affected [48]. Therefore, for some SSD patients a specific program option was developed to take into account both TCA and the head shadow effect. Amplification is reduced in the low frequencies to match the head shadow effect, and ensures good sound quality by limiting the roll-off [49]. As the sound processor is used primarily to improve speech understanding in noise, additional gain is provided for higher frequencies to increase the clarity of speech.

Direct Bone Conduction

Baha sound processors operate through direct bone conduction, where for conductive and mixed hearing loss, the conductive component is completely bypassed and amplification focuses solely on the cochlea loss. For SSD, Baha will transmit the sound directly from the impaired side to the good cochlea without the need for cables or occluding ear moulds common in CROS hearing aid solutions.

For conductive and mixed hearing losses, given that Baha effectively bypasses the conductive component, Baha should require less gain and at the same time provide performance superior to conventional air conduction hearing aids. A number of previous reports confirm that once the conductive component of a mixed hearing loss is greater than 30 dB, the Baha system should be considered in preference to conventional air conduction hearing aids [50–54].

For SSD, published studies consistently show that Baha performs better than CROS in terms of speech understanding in noise, and that the interference of noise is less with Baha than with a CROS system (Baha or CROS side) [29, 31, 32, 55, 56]. The latest Baha sound processors build on this knowledge and provide a number of key advantages that will provide further benefits for the patient. First, the measurement of BC Direct provides an improved measurement of TCA, thereby allowing for an improved fitting. Second, the frequency response of the Baha is restricted to the high frequencies (above 1,000 Hz) so that the focus is on overcoming the head shadow effect and less low-frequency noise will be amplified. Third, the noise reduction system detects and reduces the amplification of noise so that the effect of a noise-only signal interfering with a clean speech signal via the good ear is mitigated.

Discussion and Conclusions

Signal processing and fitting solutions have recently enabled a large and necessary leap in Baha performance. A number of studies have highlighted that this technology provides significant benefits to patients in terms of hearing performance and subjective reports of benefit [4–7, 57]. While the underlying cochlea hearing loss may be relatively minor in most cases, there remains significant opportunity for signal processing and the fitting of a Baha sound processor. Importantly, the programming of the Baha and signal processing features needs to be adapted to address the indications of conductive and mixed hearing loss and SSD.

The technological development of Baha does not end here. There are increasing opportunities to maximize the potential of the patient. Technological challenges remain with the Baha system as well as with how to provide the best possible solution for our patients. As signal processing continues to develop, the ability to develop improved signal process algorithms continues. Importantly, as we have discussed, it is not possible to immediately port these over from hearing aid applications. The listening needs and also the signal processing possibilities for bone conduction hearing are significantly different than for air conduction hearing and require their own dedicated research path.

References

1 Dun CAJ, de Wolf MJF, Wigren S, et al: Development and multi-centre clinical investigation of a novel Baha implant system. Technical and 6 month data; in 11th International Conference on Cochlear Implants and Other Implantable Auditory Technologies, Stockholm, 2010.

2 Gottlow J, Sennerby L, Rosengren A, Flynn M: An experimental evaluation of a new craniofacial implant using the rabbit tibia model. I. Histologic findings. Otol Neurotol 2010;31:832–839.

3 Sennerby L, Gottlow J, Rosengren A, Flynn M: An experimental evaluation of a new craniofacial implant using the rabbit tibia model. II. Biomechanical findings. Otol Neurotol 2010;31:840–845.

4 Flynn MC, Sadeghi A, Halvarsson G: Results of the first clinical evaluation of Cochlear™ Baha® BP100. Göteborg, Cochlear Bone Anchored Solutions, 2009.

5 Davison T, Leese D, Marley S, Johnson IJ: Clinical impressions of a new Bone Anchored Hearing Aid processor; in 2nd International Symposium on Bone Conduction Hearing – Craniofacial Osseointegration, Göteborg, June 2009.

6 Kompis M, Pfiffner F: A prospective comparative study of Baha BP100 and Baha Divino; in 11th International Conference on Cochlear Implants and Other Implantable Auditory Technologies, Stockholm, 2010.

7 Wong T, Yu J, Soo G, van Hasselt A: Will the new fully programmable sound processor Cochlear Baha BP100 provide additional benefits to subjects with conductive hearing loss and single-sided sensorineural deafness? in 7th Asia Pacific Symposium on Cochlear Implant and Related Sciences, Singapore, December 2009.
8 Stenfelt S: Advantage of using directional microphones in a Baha device: the Divino; in First International Symposium on Bone Conduction and Osseointegration. Halifax, 2007.
9 Flynn MC: Audiological concept behind the new Cochlear Baha BP100; in Technological Innovations: Otolaryngology – Head and Neck Surgery, Hong Kong, October–November 2009.
10 Hällgren M, Larsby B, Arlinger S: A Swedish version of the Hearing In Noise Test (HINT) for measurement of speech recognition. Int J Audiol 2006;45:227–237.
11 Kompis M, Krebs M, Hausler R: Speech understanding in quiet and in noise with the bone-anchored hearing aids Baha Compact and Baha Divino. Acta Otolaryngol 2007;127:829–835.
12 Bentler RA: Effectiveness of directional microphones and noise reduction schemes in hearing aids: a systematic review of the evidence. J Am Acad Audiol 2005;16:473–484.
13 Walden BE, Surr RK, Cord MT: Real-world performance of directional microphone hearing aids. Hear J 2003; 56:40–47.
14 Flynn MC: Maintaining the directional advantage in open fittings. Hear Rev 2004;11:32–36.
15 Blackmore KJ, Kernohan MD, Davison T, Johnson IJ: Bone-anchored hearing aid modified with directional microphone: do patients benefit? J Laryngol Otol 2007;121:822–825.
16 Oeding K, Valente M, Kerckhoff J: The effectiveness of the directional microphone in the Baha Divino. J Am Acad Audiol 2010;21:546–557.
17 Gifford RH, Revit LJ: Speech perception for adult cochlear implant recipients in a realistic background noise: effectiveness of preprocessing strategies and external options for improving speech recognition in noise. J Am Acad Audiol 2010;21: 441–451; quiz 87–88.
18 Blamey PJ, Fiket HJ, Steele BR: Improving speech intelligibility in background noise with an adaptive directional microphone. J Am Acad Audiol 2006;17: 519–530.
19 Bentler R, Palmer C, Mueller HG: Evaluation of a second-order directional microphone hearing aid. I. Speech perception outcomes. J Am Acad Audiol 2006;17:179–189.
20 Chung K: Challenges and recent developments in hearing aids. I. Speech understanding in noise, microphone technologies and noise reduction algorithms. Trends Amplif 2004;8:83–124.
21 Mackenzie E, Lutman ME: Speech recognition and comfort using hearing instruments with adaptive directional characteristics in asymmetric listening conditions. Ear Hear 2005;26:669–679.
22 Ricketts T, Henry P: Evaluation of an adaptive, directional-microphone hearing aid. Int J Audiol 2002;41:100–112.
23 Kuk F, Keenan D, Lau CC, Ludvigsen C: Performance of a fully adaptive directional microphone to signals presented from various azimuths. J Am Acad Audiol 2005;16:333–347.
24 Maj JB, Wouters J, Moonen M: Noise reduction results of an adaptive filtering technique for dual-microphone behind-the-ear hearing aids. Ear Hear 2004;25: 215–229.
25 Dillon H: Hearing Aids. New York, Thieme, 2001.
26 Alcantara JI, Moore AP, Kuhnel V, Launer S: Evaluation of a noise reduction system in a commercial digital hearing aid. Int J Audiol 2003;42:34–42.
27 Boymans M, Dreschler WA: Field trials using a digital hearing aid with active noise reduction and dual-microphone directionality. Audiology 2000;39: 260–268.
28 Bentler R, Wu YH, Kettel J, Hurtig R: Digital noise reduction: outcomes from laboratory and field studies. Int J Audiol 2008;47:447–460.
29 Hol MK, Bosman AJ, Snik AF, Mylanus EA, Cremers CW: Bone-anchored hearing aid in unilateral inner ear deafness: a study of 20 patients. Audiol Neurootol 2004;9:274–281.
30 Hol MK, Bosman AJ, Snik AF, Mylanus EA, Cremers CW: Bone-anchored hearing aids in unilateral inner ear deafness: an evaluation of audiometric and patient outcome measurements. Otol Neurotol 2005;26:999–1006.
31 Lin LM, Bowditch S, Anderson MJ, May B, Cox KM, Niparko JK: Amplification in the rehabilitation of unilateral deafness: speech in noise and directional hearing effects with bone-anchored hearing and contralateral routing of signal amplification. Otol Neurotol 2006;27:172–182.
32 Niparko JK, Cox KM, Lustig LR: Comparison of the bone anchored hearing aid implantable hearing device with contralateral routing of offside signal amplification in the rehabilitation of unilateral deafness. Otol Neurotol 2003; 24:73–78.
33 Chung K: Challenges and recent developments in hearing aids. II. Feedback and occlusion effect reduction strategies, laser shell manufacturing processes, and other signal processing technologies. Trends Amplif 2004;8:125–164.
34 Verstraeten N, Zarowski AJ, Somers T, Riff D, Offeciers EF: Comparison of the audiologic results obtained with the bone-anchored hearing aid attached to the headband, the testband, and to the 'snap' abutment. Otol Neurotol 2009;30: 70–75.
35 Eeg-Olofsson M, Stenfelt S, Tjellstrom A, Granstrom G: Transmission of bone-conducted sound in the human skull measured by cochlear vibrations. Int J Audiol 2008;47:761–769.
36 Nolan M, Lyon DJ: Transcranial attenuation in bone conduction audiometry. J Laryngol Otol 1981;95:597–608.
37 Gatehouse S, Naylor G, Elberling C: Linear and nonlinear hearing aid fittings. 1. Patterns of benefit. Int J Audiol 2006;45: 130–152.
38 Wood SA, Lutman ME: Relative benefits of linear analogue and advanced digital hearing aids. Int J Audiol 2004; 43:144–155.
39 Valente M, Fabry DA, Potts LG, Sandlin RE: Comparing the performance of the Widex SENSO digital hearing aid with analog hearing aids. J Am Acad Audiol 1998;9:342–360.
40 Schum D, Elberling C: DigiFocus Audiological Research Documentation. News from Oticon, 1996.
41 Schum DJ, Pogash RR: Blinded comparison of three levels of hearing aid technologies. Hear Rev 2003;10:40–43, 64–65.
42 Souza PE, Bishop RD: Improving speech audibility with wide dynamic range compression in listeners with severe sensorineural loss. Ear Hear 1999;20: 461–470.

43 Flynn MC, Davis PB, Pogash R: Multiple-channel non-linear power hearing instruments for children with severe hearing impairment: long-term follow-up. Int J Audiol 2004;43: 479–485.
44 Marriage JE, Moore BC, Stone MA, Baer T: Effects of three amplification strategies on speech perception by children with severe and profound hearing loss. Ear Hear 2005;26:35–47.
45 Lybarger SF (inventor): US Patent Application, 1944.
46 Stenfelt S, Hakansson B: Air versus bone conduction: an equal loudness investigation. Hear Res 2002;167:1–12.
47 Snyder JM: Interaural attenuation characteristics in audiometry. Laryngoscope 1973;83:1847–1855.
48 Feddersen WE, Sandel TT, Teas DC, Jeffress LA: Localization of high frequency tones. J Acoust Soc Am 1957;29: 988–991.
49 Pfiffner F, Kompis M, Flynn MC, Åsnes K, Arnold A, Stieger C: Benefits of low frequency attenuation of Baha in single sided sensorineural deafness. Ear Hear, Epub ahead of print.
50 Hol MK, Snik AF, Mylanus EA, Cremers CW: Long-term results of bone-anchored hearing aid recipients who had previously used air-conduction hearing aids. Arch Otolaryngol Head Neck Surg 2005;131:321–325.
51 Mylanus EA, Snik AF, Cremers CW: Patients' opinions of bone-anchored vs conventional hearing aids. Arch Otolaryngol Head Neck Surg 1995;121: 421–425.
52 Mylanus EA, van der Pouw KC, Snik AF, Cremers CW: Intraindividual comparison of the bone-anchored hearing aid and air-conduction hearing aids. Arch Otolaryngol Head Neck Surg 1998;124: 271–276.
53 McDermott AL, Dutt SN, Reid AP, Proops DW: An intra-individual comparison of the previous conventional hearing aid with the bone-anchored hearing aid: The Nijmegen group questionnaire. J Laryngol Otol 2002;116:15–19.
54 Flynn MC, Sadeghi A, Halvarsson G: Baha solutions for patients with severe mixed hearing loss. Cochlear Implants Int 2009;10(suppl 1):43–47.
55 Wazen JJ, Spitzer JB, Ghossaini SN, et al: Transcranial contralateral cochlear stimulation in unilateral deafness. Otolaryngol Head Neck Surg 2003;129:248–254.
56 Hol MK, Snik AF, Mylanus EA, Cremers CW: Does the bone-anchored hearing aid have a complementary effect on audiological and subjective outcomes in patients with unilateral conductive hearing loss? Audiol Neurootol 2005;10: 159–168.
57 Yu J, Soo G, Van Hasselt A, Soli S, Tong M: Comparison of hearing performance between Cochlear BP100 and a control Baha at CUHK in Hong Kong; in Technological Innovations: Otolaryngology – Head and Neck Surgery, Hong Kong, October–November 2009.

Mark C. Flynn, PhD
Cochlear Bone Anchored Solutions AB
PO Box 82
SE–435 22 Mölnlycke (Sweden)
Tel. +46 31 792 44 68, Fax +46 31 792 46 95, E-Mail mflynn@cochlear.com

Kompis M, Caversaccio M-D (eds): Implantable Bone Conduction Hearing Aids.
Adv Otorhinolaryngol. Basel, Karger, 2011, vol 71, pp 124–131

Headbands, Testbands and Softbands in Preoperative Testing and Application of Bone-Anchored Devices in Adults and Children

Andrzej J. Zarowski · Nadia Verstraeten · Thomas Somers · Daphna Riff · Erwin F. Offeciers

University ENT Department, St. Augustinus Hospital, Antwerp, Belgium

Abstract

The headbands, the testbands and the softbands are applied for coupling of the sound processors of the bone-anchored devices to the patient's head before the titanium fixture/abutment can be implanted. The bands are used for acute and/or prolonged testing of the bone-anchored devices, and are able to approximate the results of postoperative amplification. Yet, whatever the type of the band coupling, the transducers interface with the bone through a layer of skin and subcutaneous tissue that damp the transmission and decrease effective amplification. Therefore, the final hearing result with the bone-anchored device after implantation is usually better than with the sound processor attached to the headband, testband or softband, especially in the high-frequency zone. The results of our studies performed in experienced Baha Compact users quantified the magnitude of the skin damping and showed significant threshold differences for frequencies 1–4 kHz (in the range of 5–20 dB) when the Baha was coupled to the implanted fixture/abutment, as compared to the headband or the testband. These differences were also reflected in speech audiometry with the speech reception threshold improvement of approximately 4–7 dB. Suboptimal character of audiometric thresholds and speech understanding scores found during the preoperative testing period must be carefully considered in patient counseling, because such suboptimal results obtained preoperatively could demotivate the patients from using the Baha. Audiometrical results obtained with the headband and the testband are comparable; therefore, the more comfortable headband is also suitable for the preoperative audiological evaluation, especially in children.

Importance of Preoperative Evaluation of Bone-Anchored Devices

Success in application of hearing aids depends on the ratio between the severity of hearing loss and the magnitude of potential gain the hearing aid can provide in a particular patient. If the hearing loss is severe and the solution can provide substantial gain, it will most probably be well received by the patient. If, however, the potential improvement offered by the hearing aid becomes smaller, the disadvantages, such as the need for surgery, pain, discomfort, cosmetics, price, etc., begin to play a more important role.

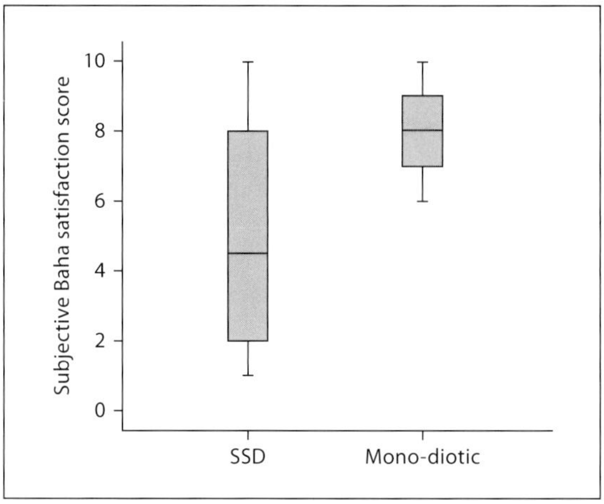

Fig. 1. Comparison of the subjective Baha satisfaction scores in 2 groups of 30 patients each with two different Baha indications: SSD and bilateral conductive hearing loss (mono-diotic application). The scores were measured on the Visual Analogue Scale (VAS) between the extreme ends: 'totally not satisfied' (score = 0) and 'extremely satisfied' (score = 10). The term 'mono-diotic' stands for a condition when one Baha is applied in a patient with bilateral conductive or mixed hearing loss. In such a situation, the monophonic input of one Baha is delivered with comparable intensity to both ears.

This can be very well seen in application of the bone-anchored devices. In relatively easy indications of bilateral aural atresia or bilateral chronic otitis, the Baha offer huge improvement and are very well accepted by the patients. In a more difficult Baha indication such as, for example, the single-sided deafness (SSD), the partial relief from the head shadow offers only a minor subjective improvement, and it is much more difficult to end up with a satisfied patient.

Figure 1 shows typical results of subjective patient satisfaction scores for 2 groups of 30 patients who received Baha at our Department for two different Baha indications: SSD (where the Baha works as a transcranial cross) and bilateral conductive or mixed hearing losses (mono-diotic application). The scores were measured on a Visual Analogue Scale between the extreme ends: 'totally not satisfied' and 'extremely satisfied'. The term 'mono-diotic' stands for a condition when one Baha is applied in a patient with bilateral conductive or mixed hearing loss and delivers monophonic input to both ears with comparable intensity.

In the classical Baha mono-diotic application, the average satisfaction scores are high and show small variability. In the SSD group, the average satisfaction scores are much lower and show much larger variability. The lower 15–25% of the SSD distribution (correlating with the satisfaction scores of 2 and less) denominate potential non-users.

In order to decrease the number of less satisfied patients and non-users, the take-home trials have been introduced. They allow the patients to evaluate the actual advantage offered by the hearing aids in daily life, what is especially important in the case of difficult indications such as SSD. In this group of our patients, introduction of at least 2-week Baha trial period significantly improved our indication setting and reduced the number of non-users and only occasional users by almost threefold.

Therefore, we find the subjective take-home trial crucial for patient counseling. Such a take-home trial is easy to perform with the classical hearing aids, yet it is much less obvious in the case of bone-anchored devices. Since it is impossible to only temporarily anchor a fixture in the bone, other solutions must be used. Historically, first the test rod and later the testband and the headband were developed in order to demonstrate the working of the device and to approximate the characteristics of postoperative amplification.

The headband has also been used as a temporary solution in small children who do not have sufficient thickness of the skull bones to allow implantation of the titanium fixture. Although the headband has been useful for many children, it often proved difficult to wear due to discomfort and difficulties with keeping the headband in place especially in babies. To solve this problem a softband has been introduced in 2003.

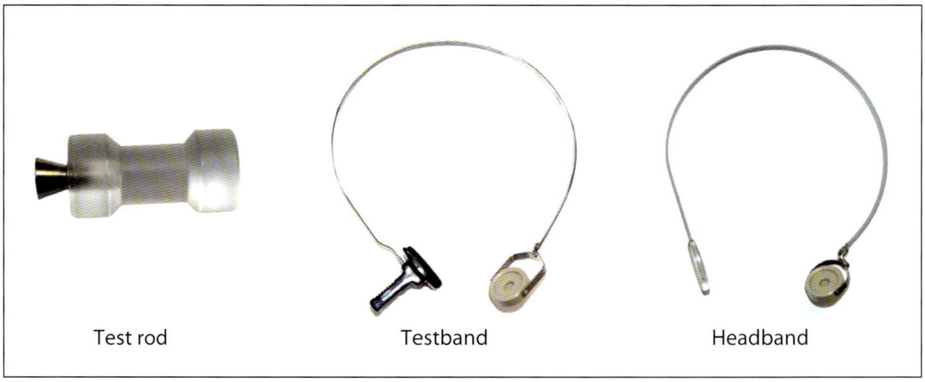

Fig. 2. Photographs showing the test rod, the testband and the headband.

Test Rod, Headband, Testband and Softband

The test rod (fig. 2) has been designed for short demonstrations of the Baha amplification in the consultation room. After coupling to the Baha device, the patient was asked to hold the test rod between the teeth and to close the lips over the rod. In this situation, the vibration was transmitted to the inner ears directly through the teeth and the bones of the skull. The test rod had an advantage of direct coupling to the bone but suffered from major disadvantages, such as increased distance to the inner ear or difficulty and impractical aspects of audiological testing. For these reasons, the test rod has been replaced by the testband.

The testband has a form of a diadem that consists of a steel spring band with attached disk connector for the Baha (fig. 2). The disk connector is placed on the mastoid, at the position of expected implantation of the titanium fixture. The testband has a tight fit to the skull and exerts relatively high pressure on the skin. This high contact force should theoretically warrant optimal sound transmission, although according to Hodgetts et al. [1] the influence of the variation in the applied contact force (pressure) on the Baha output levels is only limited, and does not exceed 3 dB.

The testband is used for acute audiometrical testing. The results of tonal liminar audiometry and speech audiometry obtained with the Baha attached to the testband aid the physician in patient counseling. These results are also often used as a gold standard for comparison with the results obtained with implantable hearing aids. Due to unpleasant pressure and pain caused by the tight fitting of the testband, the audiological examinations should not last for more than 1–2 h.

The headband (fig. 2) is very similar to the testband except for the synthetic material that replaced the steel spring band. The pressure exerted by the headband is much less than in the case of the testband, and it is suitable for long-term testing. The headband allows the patient to experience the Baha amplification during the 2-week trial period before the definitive titanium fixture is implanted in the bone.

As mentioned above, in small children the headband has been replaced by the softband. The softband (fig. 3) is an elastic band adjustable in length in order to fit the size of the baby's head. Sewn into the band, there is a plastic connector disk for coupling of the Baha sound processor. The connector disk is pressed against the skin behind the ear through the pressure from the band. This pressure is comparable to the pressure exerted by the headband. The band can be turned so that the disk is not always in the same position thus avoiding discomfort to the child. There exist

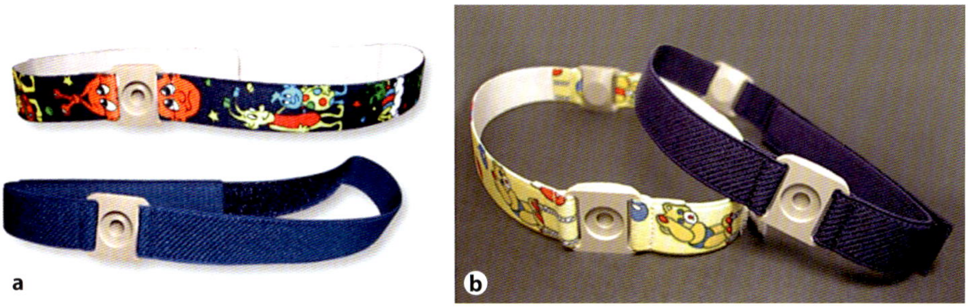

Fig. 3. The unilateral softbands (**a**) and the bilateral softbands (**b**).

also softbands with 2 connector disks suitable for bilateral Baha application (fig. 3).

Skin Damping

Whatever the type of the band coupling, be it the testband, the headband or the softband, the Baha interfaces with the bone through a layer of skin and subcutaneous tissue that damp the transmission and decrease effective amplification [2]. Therefore, the final hearing result with the Baha after implantation is usually better than with the Baha attached to the headband, the testband or the soft band, especially in the high-frequency zone. This influences not only the pure tone thresholds but also the results of speech audiometry and can be very important for the clinical decision making.

The effect of the skin damping has been evaluated in a few studies comparing the transfer functions and the speech understanding results of the Baha with the results obtained with the conventional bone conduction (BC) hearing aids that also – as in the case of the headband – interface to the bone through the skin. These studies show differences in the transfer functions at high frequencies and also a better speech understanding in favor of the percutaneous Baha transmission [3–5]. The study of Hakansson et al. [6] showed differences in acceleration levels at hearing thresholds between the direct (percutaneous) and conventional (transcutaneous) BC in a group of 7 patients. Differences between 16 and 28 dB were found for frequencies 250 Hz to 6 kHz. This study was performed with the Oticon vibrator coupled to an accelerometer fixed to the skull by a steel spring. However, the above-mentioned literature data are not fully relevant for comparison with the Baha because of significantly different resonance frequency characteristics of the Baha and the classical BC hearing aids or audiometric vibrators [5].

At our Department [7], we looked at the magnitude of the skin damping in an experimental setting involving 14 experienced adult Baha patients with bilateral air-bone gap larger or equal to 40 dB. In these patients, the differences in free field (FF) audiometric thresholds were measured between the condition when a Baha Compact was coupled to the implanted fixture/abutment versus the Baha attached to the testband and positioned as close to the abutment as possible without touching it. In both conditions, the volume control of the Baha was fixed at the same position.

As shown in figure 4, median audiometric thresholds for frequencies 1–4 kHz were between 5 and 20 dB better with the Baha coupled to the fixture/abutment than with the Baha attached to the testband. These median differences were statistically significant with $p < 0.05$ in the Wilcoxon signed rank test. For frequencies 125–500 Hz, the

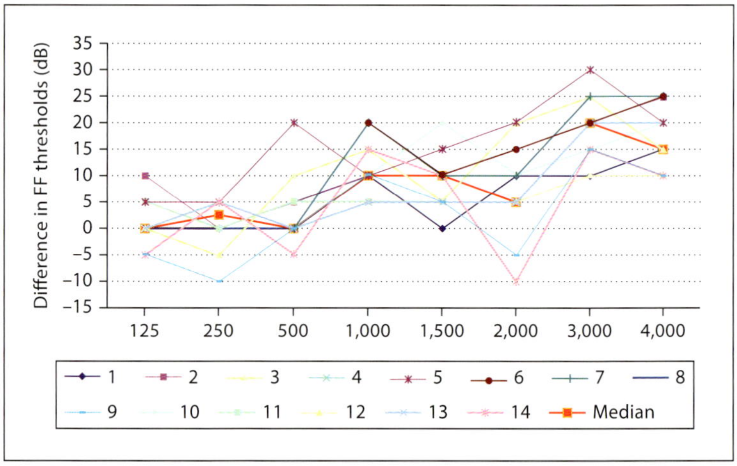

Fig. 4. Individual (14 patients) and median differences in FF thresholds between the Baha Compact attached to the implanted fixture/abutment vs. the Baha Compact coupled to the testband (volume control fixed at the constant value). This test situation quantifies the amount of damping through the skin.

median differences were close to zero and were not significant, neither statistically nor clinically.

Knowledge of the magnitude of the skin damping will allow us to make adequate predictions for the postoperative thresholds in Baha patients. It will also improve evaluation of implantable direct drive hearing aids. Audiological results obtained with these implantable hearing aids are frequently referenced to the results obtained with a Baha on the testband, but without considering the attenuation of the skin. This leads to underestimation of the results obtained with the Baha option. Therefore, the high frequency response of implantable hearing aids may be compared to the response of the Baha coupled to the testband only when it is corrected for the skin damping effects.

Differences in the Results of Pure Tone and Speech Audiometry Obtained with the Testband, the Headband and the Implanted Fixture/Abutment

We measured the intrapatient differences in the results of pure tone and speech audiometry in 3 different test conditions: with the Baha coupled to the headband, to the testband or to the implanted fixture/abutment [7]. For speech audiometry, Dutch monosyllabic adult lists (NVA) were used and the phonemic scores were measured. The tests were performed in 10 experienced adult Baha Compact users and the patients were allowed to set the Baha volume control to the most comfortable level. The results obtained with the Baha coupled to the headband correspond to the take-home Baha trial. The results with the Baha attached to the testband correspond to the situation of the clinical preoperative testing.

Figure 5 shows the median results of FF tonal audiometry obtained in each of the 3 conditions. Presentation of the median FF thresholds together with the median nonaided air conduction (AC) and BC hearing thresholds of the tested patients gives an idea of the functional gain of the Baha (defined as the difference between the postoperative FF thresholds with the Baha and the preoperative BC thresholds) for each of the conditions. For frequencies up to 500 Hz, there has been no difference measured between the FF thresholds obtained with the Baha attached to the implanted fixture/abutment and the Baha attached to the testband or the headband. For the frequencies of 1 kHz and above, the Baha coupled to the implanted fixture/abutment showed better thresholds than

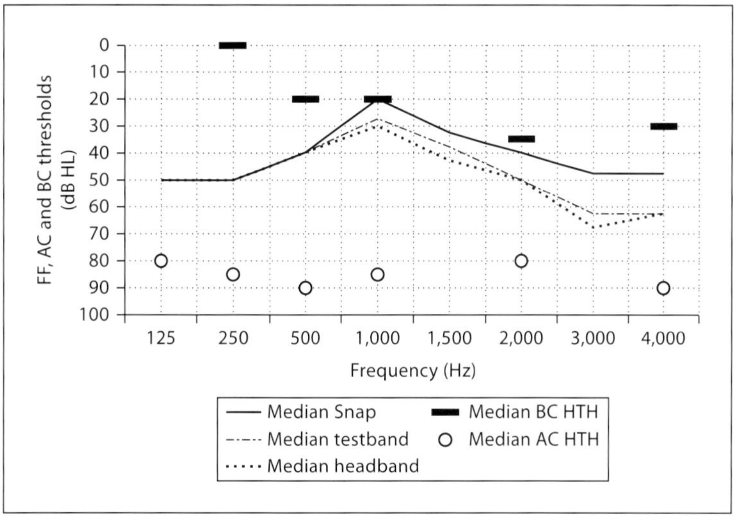

Fig. 5. Summary of the median FF thresholds for each of the 3 test conditions (with the Baha coupled to the headband, to the testband or to the implanted fixture/abutment). In all these conditions, the volume control of the Baha was set to the maximum comfortable level. Presentation of the median FF thresholds together with the median non-aided air conduction hearing thresholds (AC HTH) and the BC hearing thresholds (BC HTH) gives an idea of the functional gain of the Baha Compact for each of the 3 conditions. The thresholds measured for the Baha attached to the implanted fixture/abutment are significantly better than for the headband or the testband; however, the differences are present only at high frequencies (1–4 kHz). No significant differences have been found between the FF thresholds measured with the headband and the testband.

the Baha attached to the testband or the headband. These median differences ranged from 5 to 20 dB and were significant (Wilcoxon signed rank test, $p < 0.05$). In general, except for the resonance peaks, the higher the frequency the larger the effect of the skin damping was observed and the larger the difference between the FF thresholds.

No significant differences in FF thresholds were found between the headband and the testband, even though it could have been expected that the testband, exerting much higher force on the skull than the headband, would result in better coupling of the Baha vibration to the skull and better audiometrical results. This could not be statistically confirmed by this study, what remains in good agreement with the results of Hodgetts et al. [1].

Differences observed in pure tone audiometry have also been reflected in the results of speech audiometry. The best speech reception threshold (SRT) scores were obtained for the Baha coupled to the implanted fixture/abutment, then for the testband and the headband. The median difference in SRT between the Baha coupled to the fixture/abutment and the Baha attached to the headband was 7 dB ($p < 0.05$ at the Wilcoxon signed rank test). The median difference in SRT between the Baha coupled to the fixture/abutment and the Baha attached to the testband was 4 dB and was close to the significance level ($p = 0.059$). The

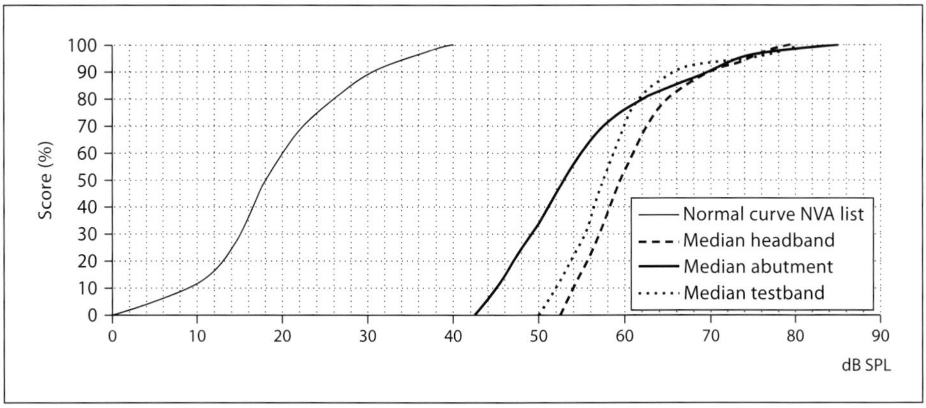

Fig. 6. Summary of the median results of speech audiometry for 3 test conditions (with the Baha coupled to the headband, to the testband or to the implanted fixture/abutment). The Dutch adult monosyllabic word lists (NVA lists) were used for speech audiometry and the phonemic scores were measured. The displayed curves were smoothened by polynominal fit. The best SRT scores were obtained for the implanted abutment, then for the testband and the headband. The differences in SRT between the headband and the testband were not significant.

improvement in SRT (4–7 dB) agrees well with approximately 6 dB improvement in the averaged middle frequency pure tone thresholds (pure-tone averages of 0.5, 1 and 2 kHz). The differences in SRT between the headband and the testband were not significant.

Discussion and Conclusions

Differences in audiometric thresholds and speech understanding scores found between the preoperative test, the take-home situations and the final postoperative results are significant at high frequencies and must be considered during patient counseling. These differences amount to 5–20 dB for the frequencies 1–4 kHz, and are also reflected in the speech audiometry with improvement in SRT of approximately 4–7 dB when the Baha is attached to the implanted fixture/abutment, compared to the headband or the testband. The 4–7 dB difference in SRT translates into approximately 20–40% difference in speech understanding scores (fig. 6). This means that in test conditions speech discrimination is far from optimal. Also the fact that only high frequencies are damped and the low frequencies are not can have additional deleterious effect in noisy environments. If we do not make up for the suboptimal results obtained during the preoperative testing and/or the take-home trial, these factors might demotivate patients from using the Baha, whilst these patients, if implanted, could potentially benefit from Baha amplification.

Therefore, we suggest that during the preoperative speech audiometry tests, a correction factor of 4–7 dB is applied to the intensity of the speech signal in order to obtain a more realistic prediction of the final result in Baha candidates with bilateral conductive/mixed losses. Another suggestion is to use a Baha with a higher force output during the preoperative testing. Therefore, for testing of the Baha Divino, BP100 or the Ponto-Pro devices, the Baha Intenso or a corresponding high-power Ponto system could be used (provided accurate adjustment of the tone setting and damping of the low frequencies). Such approach could partially compensate for the high frequency attenuation caused by the skin.

Audiometrical results obtained with the headband and the testband are comparable; therefore, the more comfortable headband is also suitable for the preoperative audiological evaluation. This might be especially important for testing children.

Concerning the softband and its use in small children, there exist no literature data on the differences in thresholds and speech discrimination scores between the softband and the Baha attached to the implanted fixture/abutment. On one hand, the pressure at the level of the disc connector should be comparable to the pressure exerted by the headband, and as such the softband should produce similar audiological results as the headband. Yet, due to the adjustable length of the softband, the tightness of fitting and the contact force are difficult to control. Also the thickness of the skin in small children is less than in adults, which could also influence the transfer function. Therefore, even though the above-mentioned study of Hodgetts et al. [1] found only minimal differences in the audiometrical thresholds due to the variations in the applied contact force (not exceeding 3 dB) and the study of Mylanus et al. [8] found no relation between the thickness of the skin and the difference in averaged thresholds for transcutaneously coupled vibrators in the frequency range of 250 Hz to 4 kHz, the exact data for the softband are lacking and further formal evaluation would be interesting.

References

1 Hodgetts WE, Scollie SD, Swain R: Effects of applied contact force and volume control setting on output force levels of the Baha softband. Int J Audiol 2006;45:301–308.

2 Hakansson B, Tjellstrom A, Rosenhall U: Hearing thresholds with direct bone conduction versus conventional bone conduction. Scand Audiol 1984;13:3–13.

3 van der Pouw CTM, Snik AFM, Cremers CWRJ: The Baha HC200/300 in comparison with conventional bone conduction hearing aids. Clin Otolaryngol Allied Sci 1999;24:171–176.

4 Browing GG, Stuart Gatehouse S: Estimation of the benefit of bone-anchored hearing aids. Ann Otol Rhinol Laryngol 1994;103:872–878.

5 Hakansson B, Carlsson P, Tjellström A, Lidén G: The bone-anchored hearing aid: principal design and audiometric results. Ear Nose Throat J 1994;73: 670–675.

6 Hakansson B, Tjellstrom A, Rosenhall U: Acceleration levels at hearing threshold with direct bone conduction versus conventional bone conduction. Acta Otolaryngol 1985;100:240–252.

7 Verstraeten N, Zarowski AJ, Somers T, Riff D, Offeciers EF: Comparison of the audiologic results obtained with the bone-anchored hearing aid attached to the headband, the testband, and to the 'Snap' abutment. Otol Neurotol 2009;30: 70–75.

8 Mylanus EA, Snik AF, Cremers CW: Influence of the thickness of the skin and subcutaneous tissue covering the mastoid on bone-conduction thresholds obtained transcutaneously versus percutaneously. Scand Audiol 1994;23: 201–203.

Dr. Andrzej Zarowski
University ENT Department, St. Augustinus Hospital
Oosterveldlaan 24
BE–2610 Antwerp (Belgium)
Tel. +32 3 443 36 14, Fax +32 3 443 36 11, E-Mail Andrzej.Zarowski@GZA.be

Kompis M, Caversaccio M-D (eds): Implantable Bone Conduction Hearing Aids.
Adv Otorhinolaryngol. Basel, Karger, 2011, vol 71, pp 132–139

Bone-Anchored Hearing Aids versus Conventional Hearing Aids

Rupan Banga · Rebecca Lawrence · Andrew Reid · Ann-Louise McDermott

Departments of Paediatric Audiology and Paediatric Otolaryngology, The Birmingham Children's Hospital, Steelhouse Lane, Birmingham, UK

Abstract

Hearing amplification technology has been evolving since the 19th century. Currently in most audiology departments, the mainstay of hearing rehabilitation is performed with conventional air and bone conduction aids. These are cost-effective, non-invasive hearing aids but are not without their drawbacks. This chapter explores the advantages and disadvantages of conventional hearing aids compared with the bone-anchored hearing aids. Although the bone-anchored hearing aids are a more expensive invasive option, there is increasing evidence that the benefits outweigh the disadvantages. Users report improved quality of life, health status and audiological rehabilitation.

Hearing amplification is noted as far back as prehistoric times with animal horns used to amplify speech. At the beginning of the 19th century, early hearing aids in the form of ear trumpets were used to direct sound at hearing-impaired individuals [1].

In 1876, the first bone conduction (BC) hearing aid was described by Prof. Paladino at the University of Naples. It consisted of a metal rod; one end was placed on the speaker's larynx and the other end against the teeth or mastoid of the listener. The device was called a Fonifero [2]. This still required a direct physical link between the speaker and the listener in order to function. See figure 2 in the chapter by Mudry and Tjellström [this vol.].

In the 1920s with the advent of electricity and with Alexander Graham Bell's work on the telephone, hearing aid technology had advanced and the electric hearing aid had become commercially available [3]. In the 1960s, the transistor technology made the 'behind the ear' air conduction (AC) hearing aids a reality [1].

For those patients requiring a bone conductor hearing aid, there was an electromagnetic vibrator designed to press against the mastoid by a tight steel headband. This was uncomfortable and very unsightly. The hearing spectacles were considered a more cosmetic alternative (fig. 1).

Modern day conventional hearing aids have three main components:

A microphone that converts sound energy to electrical energy, an amplifier and a receiver to convert the modified and amplified electrical impulses back into to sound.

These conventional hearing aids can be separated into two types, those that work by AC and those that work by BC.

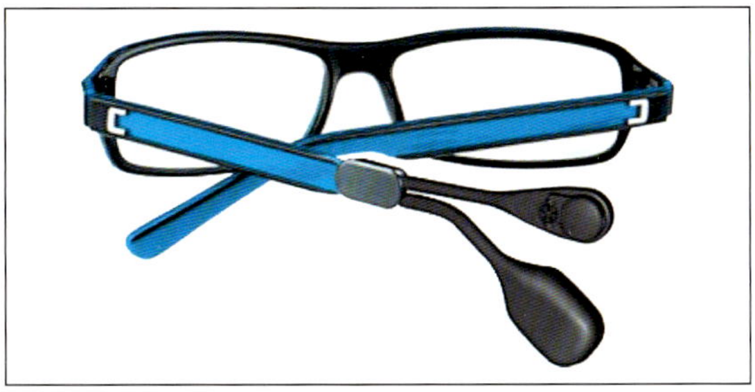

Fig. 1. The hearing spectacle. http://www.thedeafblog.co.uk/2009/03/hidden_hearings_spectacle_hear.html.

This chapter aims to discuss the merits of both conventional AC and BC hearing aids and compare them with the bone-anchored hearing aid.

Conventional Air Conduction Devices

An AC device uses an ear mould or a 'dome' coupling to deliver amplified sound directly into the ear canal. The receiver and microphone are traditionally worn behind the ear and coupled to the ear mould by a small length of plastic tubing (fig. 2). Smaller 'in the ear' AC hearing aids are also available. A bespoke device is made to incorporate the receiver and microphone in a plastic shell which is fitted directly into the conchal bowl or the ear canal, making it almost invisible.

There are also body-worn versions, where the microphone is worn on the clothing and the receiver is attached to the ear mould. The receiver and microphone are attached to each other by a wire (fig. 3).

Conventional Bone Conduction Devices

With the BC aids, the receiver is attached to an oscillator that vibrates. BC hearing aids may be either a body-worn or ear level device (incorporating the microphone and amplifier) attached to an oscillator that vibrates in relation to the sounds entering the

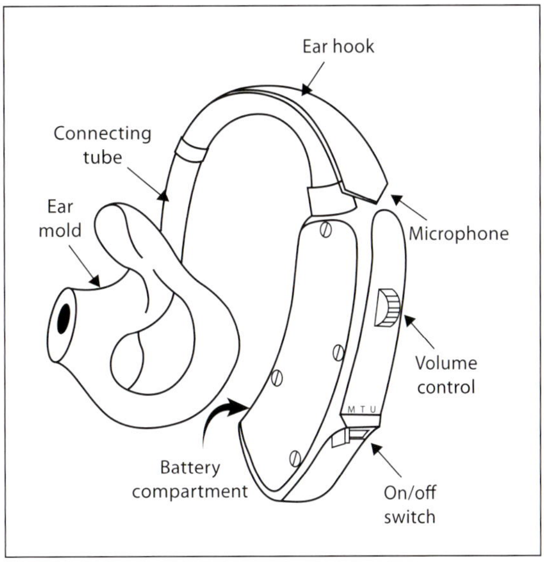

Fig. 2. Behind the ear AC hearing aid. http://www.bc-childrens.ca/Services/ClinicalDiagnosticFamilyServices/Audiology/Forfamilies/hearingaids.htm.

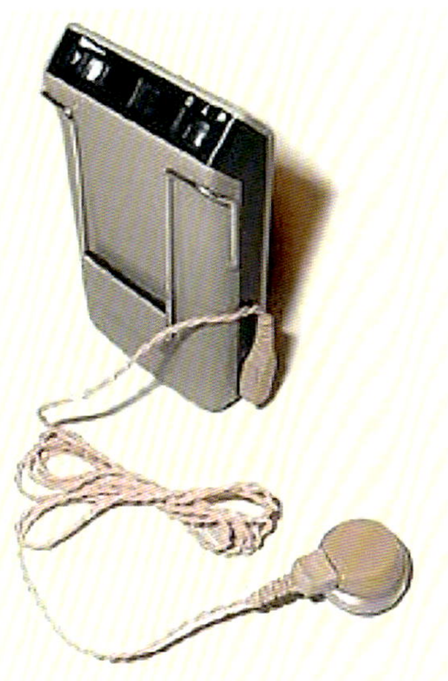

Fig. 3. Body-worn hearing aid. http://www.voonradio.com/body.php.

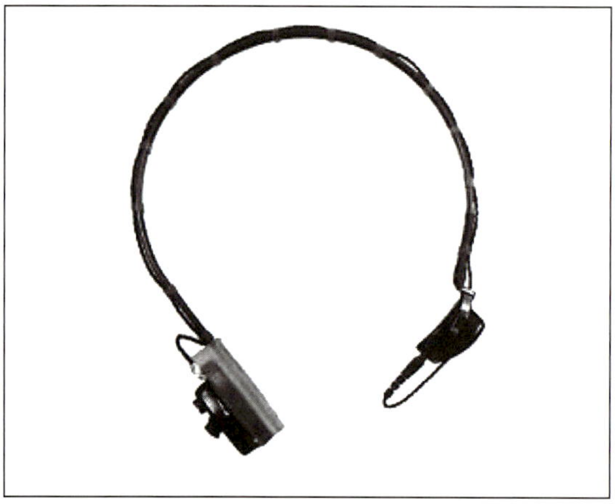

Fig. 4. BC hearing aid. http://boingboing.net/2006/01/09/musician-requests-tr.html.

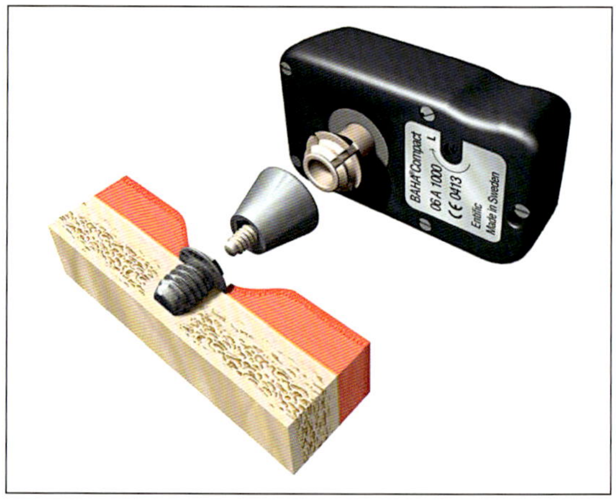

Fig. 5. Baha. http://www.ent.uci.edu/BAHA.htm.

hearing aid microphone. The oscillator is placed against the skin overlying the mastoid process and is held in place either by a sprung headband, or it is worn on an elastic headband (such as a sports sweatband or the Baha Softband®). In the latter case, the bone oscillator and the hearing aid are held in place by Velcro pads that attach to the headband.

In the ear level device, the hearing aid is attached to one side of the headband and the oscillator to the other. A wire is threaded over the headband to connect the hearing aid to the oscillator (fig. 4). In patients with poorer BC thresholds, a more powerful body-worn device can be used.

BC aids are most commonly indicated where an AC aid is not suitable, for example in patients with chronic otitis externa, congenital ear canal atresia or in patients with anatomical abnormalities following mastoid surgery.

Bone-Anchored Hearing Aids

In 1980, Tjellström and his team described the combination of osseointegration and direct BC with a hearing aid [4]. In 1987, the first semi-implantable BC hearing aids became commercially available [4–6]. They consisted of a titanium fixture and abutment secured to the skull by osseointegration. The sound processor attached directly to the abutment (fig. 5).

The percutaneous bone-anchored hearing aid (Baha®) has since proven to be an effective method of rehabilitation for patients with both unilateral and bilateral conductive and mixed hearing loss [7, 8]. A summary of the evidence regarding bone anchored and conventional hearing aids can be found in table 1.

Advantages of Baha versus Bone Conduction and Air Conduction Hearing Aids

Sound Quality

Compared to the Baha, sound clarity is compromised using a conventional BC device, particularly at the low and high frequencies. This is a result of sound dissipating within the hair, skin and muscle tissue before reaching the bone of the mastoid.

Christensen et al. [9] found a statistically significant audiological improvement in children with a Baha compared with traditional BC aids. Interestingly, they found that there was no significant difference in these children between the Baha Softband and the implanted Baha. Studies from

Table 1. Summary of the evidence for Baha

Reference	First author	Methods	Results
[7]	Mylanus	Questionnaire	Improved speech in quiet and noise and improved sound quality with Baha
[9]	Christensen	Audiometric tests	Improved functional gain over BC aids
[10]	McDermott	Nijmegen questionnaire	Baha better in all audiological and patient respects
[11]	Mylanus	Questionnaire and audiometric tests	Small improvement with speech in noise with the Baha but majority of patients preferred Baha
[12]	Bonding	Audiological audit	Baha superior to BC and AC aids, but speech discrimination in noise was the same with Baha, AC and BC
[13]	Oeding	Hearing in Noise Test (HINT) and abbreviated profile of hearing aid benefit questionnaire (APHAB)	Directional microphone was much better in Baha for Speech in Noise Test
[15]	Hol	Audiometric tests	Better speech in noise
[16]	Hol	APHAB	Improved speech in noise with Baha as a CROS aid. Significant benefit with the APHAB
[17]	Lin	Subjective benefit questionnaire, HINT	Benefit for most patients with a degree of SNHL with Baha
[18]	Hol	Audiological tests, Directional hearing questionnaire, APHAB	Benefit with Baha, BC and AC
[19]	Bosman	Audiological tests	Directional hearing and speech in noise improved with Baha
[20]	Hol	Audiological tests	Baha Softband as good as other aids
[21]	Doshi	Glasgow children's benefit inventory (GCBI)	Improved quality of life with Baha
[22]	Snik	Audiological tests, questionnaire	Baha was better than previous conventional aids
[23]	Hol	Aided free field speech in noise and quiet	Improved speech in quiet and speech localisation
[26]	De Wolf	Glasgow benefit inventory (GBI), APHAB, Nijmegen cochlear implant questionnaire, Hearing handicap inventory for the elderly	Better quality of life
[27]	Hol	6-item short form health survey, EuroQol-5D, Hearing handicap and disability inventory	Improved quality of life

Table 1. Continued

Reference	First author	Methods	Results
[28]	Kunst	GCBI, Listening inventory for education questionnaire	Subjective benefit with Baha
[30]	Dutt	GBI, Health status	Benefit with bilateral Baha and improved health status
[33]	McDermott	GCBI	Benefit with Baha

both Nijmegen and Birmingham have also shown that patients report a subjective improvement in sound quality using the Baha compared with traditional BC aids [7, 10, 11].

Better speech recognition is mentioned most frequently as an advantage of Baha over conventional hearing aids, particularly in noisy surroundings [7]. Two smaller studies reported a statistically significant improvement in questionnaire results with the Baha compared to BC aids. Interestingly, this improvement was not demonstrated in the speech discrimination test on the same patients [7, 12].

With a Baha, sound bypasses the 'problem areas' – the outer and middle ear, and maximises the level and quality of sound that reaches the cochlea.

For conditions characterised by fluctuating hearing loss but stable BC thresholds (typically middle ear effusions and infection), the sound perceived from a BC device will be consistent, whereas sound perceived with an AC device will be heavily dependent on AC thresholds at the time. This creates an issue when programming the AC aids, as most fitting formulae such as Desired Sensation Level or National Acoustics Laboratory take the AC and in some cases the BC levels into account when prescribing the amount of gain needed. If these fitting formulae calculations are constantly changing, it is impossible for the AC aid to function optimally. When compared to conventional BC aids, the Baha has been shown statistically to have as much gain as a BC transducer at 500, 1,000, 2,000 and 4,000 Hz in children [9].

Sound Localisation

The ability to localise sound is severely diminished with a BC aid. The microphone may be situated on clothing or may transmit sounds from the contralateral side. This creates unwanted background noise, leading to an unnatural listening condition. Ear level Baha sound processors have the microphone on the same side, which is a more natural listening condition.

Directional microphones in conventional AC hearing aids can provide a greater signal-to-noise ratio than omnidirectional microphones to improve speech recognition in the presence of background noise. The Baha now has the advantage of directional microphones. These have been shown to provide a statistically significant improvement in speech in noise recognition [13].

The management of unilateral hearing loss has been controversial. Recent studies however have shown the efficacy of the Baha as a contralateral routing of signal (CROS) device by eliminating the head shadow effect [14–16]. In fact, Baha has been shown to provide better amplification in subjects with unilateral hearing loss than the conventional CROS aid [17, 18].

For patients with bilateral hearing loss, results have shown that directional hearing and speech recognition in noise improves significantly with a second Baha, resulting in binaural hearing [19].

Comfort

Comfort is an issue, particularly when the BC aid is worn on a sprung headband, since this delivers a degree of pressure on the skull which can be uncomfortable if worn for long periods of time. A major development in BC was the introduction of the Baha Softband. The Baha attached to an elasticised headband has proven to be a very successful, attractive and acceptable method of hearing rehabilitation for younger children [20]. Although there are still pressure and comfort issues with the Baha Softband, the position can be easily altered to a different site on the skull.

A significant advantage of the Baha is its direct attachment to the bone. This renders the device 'weightless' from the patient's perspective. There is no pressure applied to the skin or soft tissues. Our early experience from the use of Baha in children, particularly those with severe disability, suggests that this perception of 'weightlessness' may be responsible for increased use of the Baha in this subset of children [21].

Consistency is a particularly troublesome problem when using a BC hearing aid in young children. It is very difficult to prevent the bone vibrator from slipping from the mastoid process. This problem is not encountered with the Baha system.

Cosmesis
Although some BC aids can be disguised to look like hair bands or sports sweat bands, the overall appearance of the Baha is far more cosmetically acceptable that that of a BC aid. It is our experience that teenage children, particularly boys have a reluctance to wear any BC aid due to concerns regarding their self-image. These children will have the same reluctance to wear a Baha Softband/headband, but they are more accepting of the percutaneous Baha. In studies comparing the Baha with conventional aids, visibility has been a negative factor, but still considered more favourable than conventional aids [7, 10].

Practical Fitting Issues
There are practical fitting issues that disadvantage AC aids. They require an ear mould or domed coupling to be placed in the ear canal. If there is discharge present in the ear, this will inevitably block the ear mould and lead to a failure of the amplified sound to reach the ear canal. Furthermore, the presence of an infection is a contraindication for impressions to be taken of the ear for the manufacture of ear moulds.

The presence of the ear mould or domed coupling in the ear can reduce the air flow in the ear canal resulting in a moist ear canal, increasing the risk of ear infection. This in turn can lead to inconsistent use of the device. Studies have shown that patients report a decrease in the frequency of ear infections when using a Baha as compared to conventional AC hearing aids [10, 11, 22, 23].

Children require multiple mould taking as they grow to ensure that the mould is tightly fitting for best use. Cooperation in obtaining an accurate impression for the hearing aid mould can be challenging, and complications have been reported [24, 25].

Quality of Life
Subjective benefit from patients with Baha has repeatedly been shown to be improved when compared to their prior conventional aids. This benefit has been shown in children, adults, patients with learning difficulties and more recently older users [21, 26–29]. A subjective improvement in a general state of health (and hence quality of life) has been reported with both unilateral and bilateral Baha use [30]. For those patients asked to state a preference for hearing aid, the overwhelming majority prefer Baha [10].

Disadvantages of Bone-Anchored Hearing Aids

Surgery
This is an invasive procedure and carries with it both surgical and anaesthetic risks. Surgical implantation of a fixture and percutaneous abutment are necessary for attachment of the Baha sound processor. In the adult population, it is possible to perform the surgery under a local anaesthetic technique as a 'day case procedure', thus reducing the risk to the patient.

In the paediatric population, it is more common for surgery to be performed under general anaesthesia, and often two procedures are advocated 3 months apart to allow for osseointegration. In addition to this the paediatric population is a more complex group of patients with complex anaesthetic needs. A large proportion of children will have recognised syndromes, cardiac problems and other medical comorbidities, making them a challenging group to anesthetise [31].

Osseointegration Time
The sound processor is commonly fitted after a minimum of 6 weeks following surgery in adults, and invariably 3 months is allowed to elapse between first- and second-stage surgery in children [32]. These timings are intended to allow good osseointegration of the fixture and the bone. This may be longer if surgical difficulties are encountered, most commonly thin calverial bone at the time of fixture placement [33]. There is much research into the strength of osseointegration, and it is likely that these time delays to fitting the aid will reduce [34].

Soft Tissue Complications
The maintenance of the soft tissues surrounding the Baha abutment site is vitally important to prevent inflammation, infection and ultimately fixture loss [8, 33, 35–37]. In younger Baha wearers and some adults, a second person is required to ensure that the abutment site is kept clean and healthy.

Trauma
A significant number of patients, particularly children, sustain trauma to their Baha. Fortunately, the sound processor is the most common component to be damaged. Serious trauma to the abutment site is very rare, but has been reported in the literature [38, 39].

Conclusions

Conventional hearing aids provide the mainstay of hearing rehabilitation and are usually the first-line management of hearing loss. They are cost-effective and readily available to most audiology departments. The Baha is a more expensive alternative that requires an invasive procedure(s) and has potential for postoperative complications. Despite these issues, there is increasing evidence that the advantages of Baha outweigh these recognised problems, and users both adult and children report improved quality of life, health status and audiological rehabilitation.

References

1 Weir N: Otolaryngology: An Illustrated History. London, Butterworths, 1990.
2 Berger KW: Early bone conduction hearing aid devices. Arch Otolaryngol 1976; 102:315–318.
3 Owen G: The microphone, stethoscope, telephone, and artificial aids to hearing: their historical relationship. Calif Med 1939;51:196–171.
4 Tjellström A, Håkansson B, Lindström J, et al: Analysis of the mechanical impedance of bone anchored hearing aids. Acta Otolaryngol 1980;89:85–92.
5 Hakansson B, Tjellstrom A, Rosenhall U, Carlsson P: The bone anchored hearing aid: principle design and a psychoacoustical evaluation. Acta Otolaryngol 1985; 100:229–239.
6 Tjellstrom A: Osseointegrated systems and their applications in the head and neck. Am J Otolaryngol Head Neck Surg 1989;3:39–70.
7 Mylanus E, Snik A, Cremers C: Patients' opinions of bone anchored vs conventional hearing aids. Arch Otolaryngol 1995;121:421–425.
8 Tjellstrom A, Granstrom G: Long term follow up with the bone anchored hearing aid: a review of the first 100 patients between 1977 and 1985. Ear Nose Throat J 1994;73:1132–1114.
9 Christensen L, Smith-Olinde L, Kimberlain J, Richter G, Dornhoffer J: Comparison of traditional bone-conduction hearing AIDS with the Baha system. J Am Acad Audiol 2010;21:267–273.
10 McDermott A, Dutt S, Reid A, Proops D: An intra-individual comparison of the previous conventional hearing aid with the bone anchored hearing aid – the Nijmegen group questionnaire. J Laryngol Otol 2002;116:15–19.

11 Mylanus E, Van Der Pouw K, Snik A, Cremers C: Intraindividual comparison of the bone-anchored hearing aid and air-conduction hearing aids. Arch Otolaryngol Head Neck Surg 1998;124:271–276.
12 Bonding P, Holm M, Salomon G, Ahlgren P: The bone anchored hearing aid. Osseointegration and audiological effect. Acta Otolaryngol 1992;492:42–45.
13 Oeding K, Valente M, Kerckhoff J: Effectiveness of the directional microphone in the Baha Divino™. J Am Acad Audiol 2010;21:546–557.
14 Snik A, Bosman A, Mylanus E, Cremers C: Candidacy for the bone-anchored hearing aid. Audiol Neurootol 2004;9: 190–196.
15 Hol M, Kunst S, Snik A, Bosman A, Mylanus E, Cremers C: Bone anchored hearing aids in patients with acquired and congenital unilateral inner ear deafness (Baha CROS): clinical evaluation of 56 cases. Ann Otol Rhinol Laryngol 2010;119:447–454.
16 Hol M, Bosman A, Snik A, Mylanus E, Cremers C: Bone anchored hearing aid in unilateral inner ear deafness: a study of 20 patients. Audiol Neurootol 2004;9:274–281.
17 Lin L, Bowditch S, Anderson M, May B, Cox K, Niparko J: Amplification in the rehabilitation of unilateral deafness: speech in noise and directional hearing effects with bone anchored hearing and contralateral routing of signal amplification. Otol Neurotol 2006;27:172–182.
18 Hol M, Kunst S, Snik A, Cremers C: Pilot study on the effectiveness of the conventional CROS, the transcranial CROS, and the BAHA transcranial CROS in adults with unilateral inner ear deafness. Eur Arch Otorhinolaryngol 2010;267:889–896.
19 Bosman A, Snik A, Van Der Pouw K, Mylanus E, Cremers C: Audiometric evaluation of bilaterally fitted bone anchored hearing aids. Audiology 2001;40:158–167
20 Hol M, Cremers C, Coppens-Schellekens W, Snik A: The BAHA Softband. A new treatment for young children with bilateral congenital aural atresia. Int J Pediatr Otorhinolaryngol 2005;69:973–980.
21 Doshi J, McDermott A, Reid A, Proops D: The use of a bone-anchored hearing aid (Baha) in children with severe behavioural problems – the Birmingham Baha programme experience. Int J Pediatr Otorhinolaryngol 2010;74:608–610.
22 Snik A, Mylanus E, Cremers C: The bone-anchored hearing aid compared with conventional hearing aids. Audiologic results and the patients' opinions. Otolaryngol Clin North Am 1995;28:73–83.
23 Hol M, Snik A, Mylanus E, Cremers C: Long term results of BAHA recipients, previously using air conduction hearing aids. Arch Otolaryngol Head Neck Surg 2005;131:321–325.
24 Shashinder S, Tang I, Velayutham P, Rahmat O, Loganathan A: Foreign body in the middle ear, a hearing aid complication. Med J Malaysia 2008;63:267–268.
25 Awan M, Iqbal M, Sardar Z: Iatrogenic insertion of impression mould into middle ear and mastoid and its retrieval after 9 years: a case report. J Med Case Reports 2007;1:3.
26 De Wolf M, Shival M, Hol M, Mylanus E, Cremers C, Snik A: Benefit and quality of life in older bone anchored hearing aid users. Otol Neurotol 2010;31:766–722.
27 Hol M, Spath M, Krabbe P, Van Der Pouw K, Snik A, Cremers C, et al: The bone anchored hearing aid. Quality of life assessment. Arch Otolaryngol Head Neck Surg 2004;130:394–399.
28 Kunst S, Hol M, Cremers C, Mylanus E: The bone anchored hearing aid in patients with moderate mental retardation: impact and benefit assessment. Otol Neurotol 2007;28:793–797.
29 McDermott A, Williams J, Kuo M, Reid A, Proops D: Quality of life in children fitted with a bone anchored hearing aid. Otol Neurotol 2009;30:344–349.
30 Dutt S, McDermott A, Burrell S, Cooper H, Reid A, Proops D: Patient satisfaction with bilateral bone anchored hearing aids – The Birmingham experience. J Laryngol Otol 2002;116:37–46.
31 Jones S, Dickson U, Moriarty A: Anaesthesia for insertion of bone anchored hearing aids in children: a seven year audit. Anaesthesia 2001;5:777–780.
32 Wazen J, Gupta R, Ghossaini S, Spitzer J, Farrugia M, Tjellstrom A: Osseointegration timing for Baha system loading. Laryngoscope 2007;117:794–796.
33 McDermott A, Williams J, Kuo M, Reid A, Proops D: The Birmingham pediatric bone anchored hearing aid program: a 15 year experience. Otol Neurotol 2009; 30:344–349.
34 Gottlow J, Sennerby L, Rosengren A, Flynn M: An experimental evaluation of a new craniofacial implant using the rabbit tibia model. 1. Histologic findings. Otol Neurotol 2010;31:832–839.
35 Rayes R, Tjellstrom A, Granstrom G: evaluation of implant losses and skin reactions around extra oral bone anchored implants. Otolaryngol Head Neck Surg 2000;122:272–276.
36 De Wolf M, Hol M, Huygen P, Mylanus E, Cremers C: Nijmegen results with application of a bone anchored hearing aid in children: simplified surgical technique. Ann Otol Rhinol Laryngol 2008; 117:805–814.
37 Shirazi M, Marzo S, Leonetti J: Perioperative complications with the bone-anchored hearing aid. Otolaryngol Head Neck Surg 2006;134:236–239.
38 McDermott A, Barraclough J, Reid A: Trauma, unusual complications and findings with bone anchored hearing aids: report of a case and review of the literature. J Laryngol Otol 2009;123:348–350.
39 Mestfin F, Perkins N, Brook C, Foyt D, German J: Epidural hematoma after tympanomastoidectomy and bone anchored hearing aid placement. Neurosurgery 2010;65:e1451–e1453.

Rupan Banga
Department of Paediatric Otolaryngology, The Birmingham Children's Hospital
Steelhouse Lane
Birmingham, B4 6NH (UK)
Tel. +44 121 333, ext. 8123, Fax +44 1213338121, E-Mail rupan@doctors.org.uk

Kompis M, Caversaccio M-D (eds): Implantable Bone Conduction Hearing Aids.
Adv Otorhinolaryngol. Basel, Karger, 2011, vol 71, pp 140–152

The Future of Bone Conduction Hearing Devices

Bo Håkansson

Department of Signals and Systems, Chalmers University of Technology, Göteborg, Sweden

Abstract

The bone-anchored hearing aid (Baha) is today an important rehabilitation alternative for patients with mixed and conductive hearing loss and where air conduction devices should not or cannot be used. Some patients with single-sided deafness are also successfully treated with a Baha. Despite successful treatment of these patient groups, there is always a need for future improvements. First, it is well known that Baha are associated with some drawbacks related to skin infections, accidental or spontaneous loss of the bone implant, and patient refusal for treatment due to stigma. Therefore, in this chapter some alternatives to the Baha which have the potential to reduce these drawbacks are generally discussed. They all have the common feature that they do not need a permanent skin penetration. The alternatives to the Baha are: (1) improved conventional bone conduction (BC) devices, (2) devices with an implanted transducer referred to as BC implants (BCI), (3) dental-attached devices. Disregarding skin complication issues, direct BC devices like the Baha, have a superior advantage of better sound quality in the high-frequency range. How these devices might be improved in the future is also discussed. Finally, some recent advances in the development of a new BCI system will be presented, where the implanted transducer uses a non-screw attachment to a hollow recess of the temporal bone. Some preclinical studies have been performed showing that a BCI system can provide similar or higher output as compared with a Baha.

When the first patients for the bone-anchored hearing aid (Baha) were evaluated in the mid-1980s [1] conventional bone conduction (BC) hearing devices were the 'gold standard' for treatment of patients with conductive or mixed hearing loss as a result of chronic middle ear infections or congenital malformation. The primary problem with conventional BC hearing devices, headband as well as those applied with the frames of a pair of glasses is related to static pressure of about 2 N toward the skin and soft tissue needed to transmit the vibration energy. A secondary problem is related to the dampening effect of the skin that attenuates the transmission sensitivity at higher frequencies, essentially over 2 kHz. Yet another problem is related to feedback where the aerial sound is radiated from the transducer back to the microphone.

The Baha that uses a permanent skin penetration for direct access to the skull bone for inducing sound vibrations was introduced as an alternative to conventional BC devices. This type of vibration transmission obtained with the Baha is sometimes referred to as 'direct bone conduction' (DBC). DBC hearing opened possibilities for an improved rehabilitation of these patients both in terms of wearing comfort and sound quality [2, 3]. There has been a long journey, and a historic review of the technical developments of the Baha is given by Håkansson [4].

Today, the Baha is the 'gold standard' in many countries for patients with chronic middle ear diseases and congenital malformations, and who cannot use air conduction hearing aids. A summary of the current candidacy criteria, and audiological and surgical considerations of the present Baha system, is given by Hodgetts [5]. Even though there are very good long-term rehabilitation results reported with the Baha [see for example 6], there are also some known associated drawbacks.

One main drawback is related to the fact that the skin penetration site needs lifelong daily care. Some patients may acquire a skin reaction with persistent infection and may form granulation tissue that requires surgical revision or reimplantation. Also, the bone-anchored fixture can be lost spontaneously or as a result of trauma. Among ENT specialists, there have been numerous discussions about how to improve the skin conditions and minimize the severity and the rate of complications. Finally, it should be mentioned that there are a number of potential Baha patients that reject a Baha because they cannot accept a skin penetration implant for stigma reasons.

Another issue that has been requested by audiologists, ENT doctors and patients, is if the Baha ear level sound processor could be made smaller and less conspicuous, and also if a device could be constructed to have higher gain and produce higher maximum output. These are slightly contradictory demands as a stronger device usually requires a bigger transducer and also a bigger battery because of higher current consumption. The transducer, which is a unique component in the Baha system along with the implantable titanium components, thus plays a vital role in the physical size and the power output of the Baha. Over the years, the transducer has been improved in many steps [4], and in the next section it will be described how it can be further improved to meet the needs requested by patients and hearing professionals.

Already in the beginning of 1990s when the Baha system slowly became clinically accepted, our research team identified, maybe not so unexpected, that the crucial aspects for long-term success were related to the permanent penetration of the skin and the transducer performance. Before discussing how to solve or improve these aspects it may be a good idea to look on the past and the various kinds of existing developments. Many possible alternatives have been suggested, some are used today, some ideas have been abandoned and some are currently under trial.

The aim of this chapter is to describe some alternatives to improve the rehabilitation for patients with chronic ear disease, malformations and single-sided deafness (SSD), where an air conduction device is not functioning properly. Of these, the Bone Conduction Implant (BCI) project will be presented in some more detail. Although middle ear devices might be an alternative in some cases for this patient population, they will not be covered in this paper.

Past, Present and Future Bone Conduction Hearing Systems

A brief overview of possible alternatives for providing a BC hearing system will be given below. Since many terms are used to distinguish these systems, to avoid the risk of confusion an attempt to categorize these has been made in figure 1a–g.

Transcutaneous Bone Conduction – Vibrations through the Intact Skin

Conventional Skin Attachment

This is the original system referred to as the conventional BC device characterized by that the transducer housing is pressed with a constant pressure against the skin either with a headband/

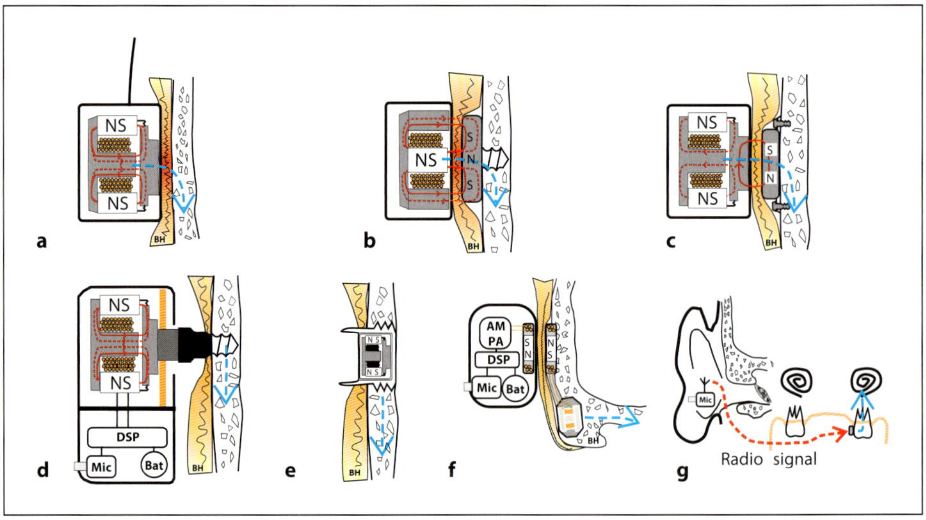

Fig. 1. Principal modalities for BC hearing systems. **Transcutaneous BC:** conventional skin attachment (**a**), the Audiant system (**b**), the Otomag system (**c**); **Percutaneous Direct BC:** the Baha system (**d**), percutaneous implanted transducer system (**e**); **Transcutaneous Direct BC:** the BCI system (**f**), in the mouth system – the SoundBite (**g**). Red lines illustrate static (solid lines) and dynamic (dashed lines) magnetic flux. Blue lines illustrate dynamic mechanic vibration transmission.

steel spring arrangement or temples of a pair of glasses, see figure 1a. As the vibrations here are transmitted through the skin and subcutaneous tissue, this mode of transduction often is referred to as transcutaneous BC.

One of the major drawbacks from a conventional BC system is, as mentioned before, related to the static pressure towards the skin. The skin will suffer from circulatory problems and sometimes irritation and eczema will develop. However, recent developments regarding this issue using a low capillary pressure design and an increased contact surface, it seems that these comfort aspects can be improved [7]. The Danish company Ortofon (http://ortofonmicrotech.com) has taken these aspects into consideration and developed a new smaller BC transducer based on the Balanced Electromagnetic Separation Transducer (BEST) principle [8], where the housing is designed to give a low capillary pressure. In this transducer, the impedance is designed to match the output impedance of the power amplifier as well as the impedance of the battery. This new design may improve the performance of conventional BC devices and may be a reasonably good low cost alternative to a Baha. One application for conventional BC, not to forget, is for the youngest children where Baha surgery is contraindicated. Finally, developments of conventional BC may be very important for a vast majority of people in many countries with a less developed health care sector, where a Baha treatment might not be afforded or is not even available.

The Audiant System

In the 1980s, the group under Jack Hough in Oklahoma developed the Xomed Audiant system [9]. This system had approximately 20 dB lower output than the Baha because the air gap needed for the generation of signal output included the skin as shown in figure 1b and that is described in more detail by Håkansson et al. [10].

The Otomag System

One interesting solution to overcome the problem with the Audiant system is suggested by Siegert [11] in his description of the Otomag system, as principally illustrated in figure 1c. In this system, there are two separate magnet systems. As far as can be understood from the limited technical information available, the transducer has its own magnet system that is optimized for maximum electromechanical transduction. The implanted magnet system is thus solely used for retention of the external transducer with the intact skin in between. It should be noted that vibrations of transducer case/plate are still transmitted by vibrations through the soft tissues (reduced to 4–5 mm) [11] and hence it is a trancutaneous BC device. As a consequence, one might expect that there is a high-frequency (HF) transmission loss of energy as in conventional BC relative to a percutaneous system. One might also expect that the skin in the contact area is under constant pressure which might cause some wearing comfort problems, and that there is a potential risk for circulatory problems if capillary issues are not considered. However, this system might be an alternative to a conventional BC system as the externally worn transducer here is more precisely attached to one and the same spot of the patient's skull bone day after day. The time independent transmission conditions might be beneficial for full adaptation in higher hearing centra in the brain. Also, this system might be more aesthetically appealing than a conventional BC device as no steel spring is needed. As usual, one has to balance these potential advantages against the more invasive surgery required and increased cost.

Percutaneous Bone Conduction – Direct Bone Conduction Systems

The Bone-Anchored Hearing Aid – the Baha System

The generic Baha system has improved the hearing conditions for a significant number of patients, and is now available from two major hearing companies, Cochlear Bone Anchored Solutions and Oticon Medical. It can be foreseen that these commercially available systems will be continuously improved and more favorably compete with other potential alternatives.

In particular, there will probably be technical solutions developed that better address the needs of different patient groups like the SSD patients. For example, a miniature transducer solution developed for the BCI system (half size compared to a typical Baha transducer) with improved HF response will offer not only a significantly smaller device, but also a significantly stronger device in the HF range (see figure 2). This HF boost will probably be very useful to patients with a HF hearing loss, but also for SSD patients where the head shadow is most pronounced at HF. The transducer developed for the BCI system is called the BCI transducer and uses a BEST as described by Håkansson [8]. Finally, the fitting procedures of the frequency response to compensate the patients' hearing loss will most likely also be improved in the future as discussed by Hodgetts et al. [12, 13]. As stated by Hodgetts, more detailed information about the patients' hearing on the implant is required. This can be done either by using built-in threshold testing functions of the digital signal processors or by using specially designed audiometric transducers and skull simulators [14].

Percutaneous-Driven Implanted Transducer

In research group at Chalmers, it was suggested already in the early 1990s that the Baha system could be potentially improved by implanting the transducer. To address the size issue, it was therefore suggested by Håkansson and Carlsson [15] that the transducer and the whole audio processor could be miniaturized and placed in the titanium screw and abutment (see figure 3a).

One such transducer was developed, but it was found to have a too low output power at low frequencies due to size issues. In this design, the fixture and abutment also needed an enlarged diameter that might increase the complication rates related to skin penetration and osseointegration,

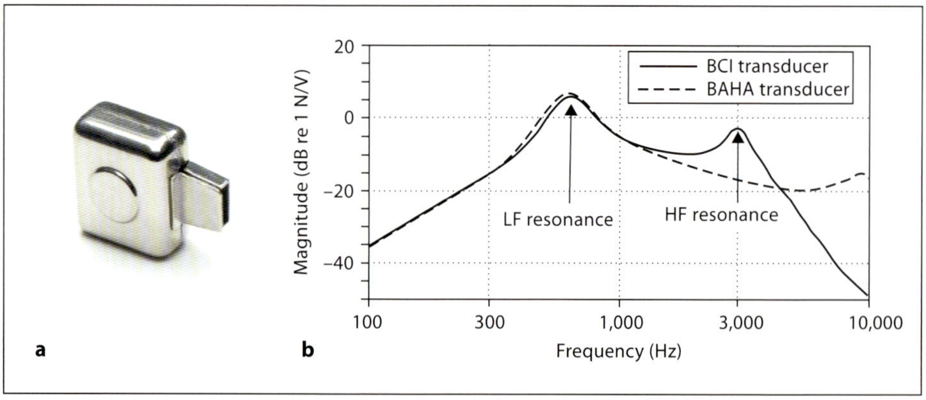

Fig. 2. The BCI transducer (**a**) has a small size and a high frequency (HF) resonance (**b**) that might be beneficial to SSD patients.

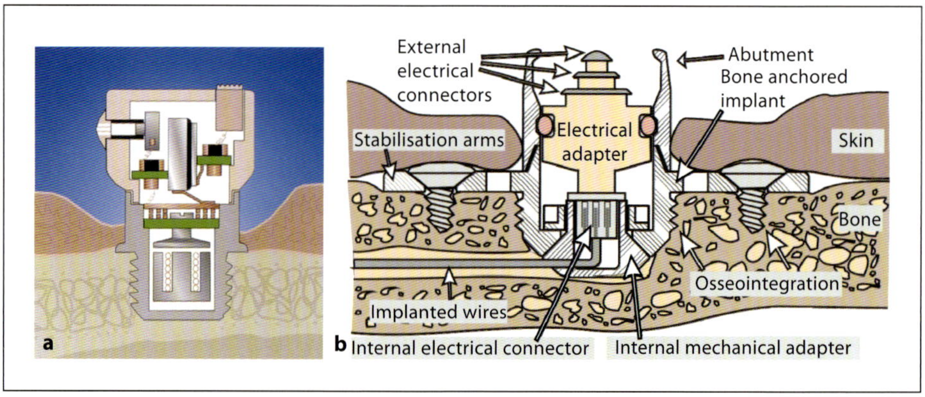

Fig. 3. A previously suggested solution where the transducer is placed in the bone-anchored fixture and abutment (**a**) or permanently implanted in the skull bone driven via a percutaneous electrical coupling (**b**).

which actually was the main reason why this idea was abandoned. In order to improve the situation, it was suggested to use a percutaneous electrical coupling [16] which directly could drive a transducer embedded in the temporal bone (see figure 3b). Definitely, such a system would be very powerful, and the external unit would be much smaller as it does not need to contain a transducer and its suspensions. However, looking into the experience from other attempts using permanent percutaneous electrical couplings to the body, there is potential risk for bacteria to enter along the bony canal containing the implanted wires to the transducer. This increased risk of complications might be acceptable, at least for the subgroup of patients that have severe sensorineural hearing loss where the Baha does not help. This idea was however abandoned as this potential

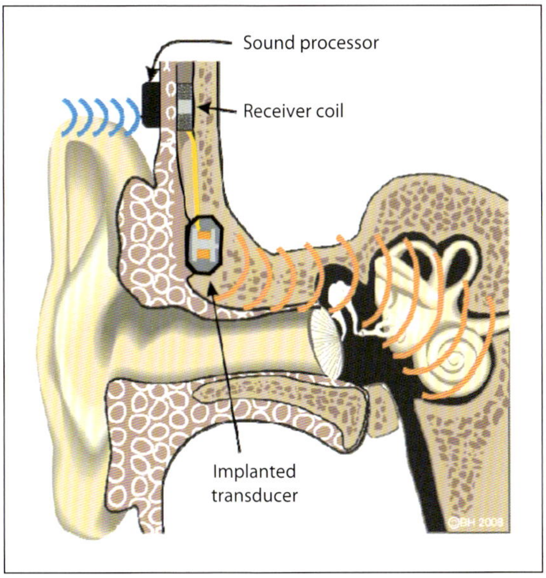

Fig. 4. Principal design of a generic transcutaneous DBC device with an implanted transducer. The sound signal is processed by the external audio processor and then transmitted by an induction link to a receiver coil that is connected to the transducer. The retention of the external device is obtained by magnets placed in the center of transmitting and receiving coils.

group of patients was too small and the risks were deemed as too high.

Transcutaneous Direct Bone Conduction
Implanted Transducer – The BCI System

A principal design of a transcutaneous DBC system with an implanted transducer is shown in figure 4. The generic feature of these systems is that the skin is kept intact, and it is the sound signal that is transmitted transcutaneously by a magnetic induction system from the external processor to the implanted transducer that is attached directly to the skull bone. Hence, it is the electric/magnetic signal that is transmitted transcutaneously (not the vibration), and the vibrations are still induced directly to the skull bone like in the Baha.

This project was started at Chalmers more than 10 years ago, and is called and referred to in what follows as the BCI system. An alternative notation of this type of system could be a transcutaneous Baha 'T-Baha' as opposed to the percutaneous bone anchored hearing aid 'P-Baha'. In principle, a BCI system can have an active or a passive drive of the implanted transducer. In an active drive system, not only the signal is transmitted, but also the electric power to supply the implanted active circuits, like in cochlear implants. In the passive drive systems, the modulated signal is transmitted, and then after demodulation it drives the transducer directly. An active drive system will be more complex than a passive system, but it may be possible to drive a higher current into the transducer that way. However, if the power is sufficient in terms of hearing level produced then it is an advantage to have a passive system as it will be less complex, more reliable and cheaper.

Obvious technical challenges with this type of system are related to (1) placement and type of attachment of the implanted transducer; (2) design of the implanted transducer; (3) design of the induction link. When we started to investigate the viability of such a system more than 10 years ago, there was some skepticism among professionals stating that this system will suffer from 'losing too much power in the induction link', 'difficulties to screw attach the transducer' and 'vulnerability and too big a size of the implanted transducer'. Some skepticism in an early phase may be healthy, and the author remembers that the Baha project during the first 10 years was regarded as weird, and many professionals had comments like 'how can anyone accept a screw through the skin', 'there will be a lot of infections', 'I don't believe this will work outside Gothenburg', etc. Facing this reluctance can be positive as it drives the motivation to prove that they were wrong. With the BCI, it was a little bit the same to start with but also very different. Nowadays, everyone seems to believe that this system principally will work even if we still have not shown that it works on a living patient. This optimism might be realistic as it is based on several preclinical studies [17–19] addressing different challenges, where the results look promising. Today (fall 2010) many hearing implant companies have announced, at least informally, that they have ongoing development projects towards a BCI device. This diversity of ongoing projects might lead to the development of slightly different technical solutions. In this chapter, the solution under development at Chalmers in collaboration with SU Sahlgrenska – the BCI system – will be described in some more detail below.

In the Mouth Bone Conduction Systems –
The SoundBite System

It is well known that BC sound can be induced by the transducer attached to the teeth. Already Beethoven held a wooden baton between his teeth and pressed it to his piano to listen to the notes. Also, a significant part of the own voice is heard via the teeth and jaw [20], so this route is definitely viable for transmission of bone-conducted sound. In fact, in the preclinical assessment of a potential Baha patient, a bite bar is used to estimate the chances for a successful treatment [21].

The idea to attach the transducer to the teeth for long-term hearing rehabilitation has been suggested by several research groups over the years. The major advantage with a solution of this kind compared with other DBC systems is that it is completely noninvasive. Several companies have announced that they have developed this idea further, for example Sonitus Medical (http://www.sonitusmedical.com). Their SoundBite system consists of a transducer that is applied to the upper left or right back teeth, principally illustrated in figure 1g. It should also be noted that the sound here has to be picked up by an external microphone, preferably worn behind the ear as also illustrated in figure 1g. This microphone should then transmit the sound wirelessly to the internal device attached to the teeth. Initial evaluations of this system have been made by Popelka et al. [22].

Whereas this idea from an electroacoustical point of view will work, one might be wondering how convenient it will be to wear the device in the mouth during one normal day. However, some inconvenience should be balanced against hearing benefits and alternative options that might involve surgery. Future clinical studies will tell how this turns out. This device is currently only available for investigational use to support an initial filing for FDA 510(k) clearance to treat SSD. Future intention is, according to the company, to extend the indications to conductive and mixed hearing loss. For SSD patients, this device may from an acoustical point of view be a good alternative as these patients only need HF gain to overcome the head shadow effect, and in that frequency range the transducer can be designed to consume less power. If this device should be aimed at those having conductive and mixed hearing loss, there might be a power issue at low frequencies. The SoundBite transducer has a relative low power output below 1 kHz as compared to Baha and BCI systems [see fig. 2 in 22].

The Bone Conduction Implant

This section is a summary of the results obtained with the transcutaneous BCI which were published by Håkansson et al. [18]. However, most of the figures of the BCI components are new and there are some updates that reflect recent developments. The structure will follow the listed 'technical challenges' with the BCI in the previous paragraph.

Placement and Type of Attachment of the Implanted Transducer

One challenge is to decide how to attach the transducer casing to the temporal bone for efficient long-term vibration transmission. From the Baha and middle ear projects, it can be learned that the system should technically be as simple as possible and that the surgery procedure should be as simple and safe as possible.

As the interior of the temporal bone is composed by spongious bone with frequent air cells, osseointegration might be jeopardized if a conventional screw

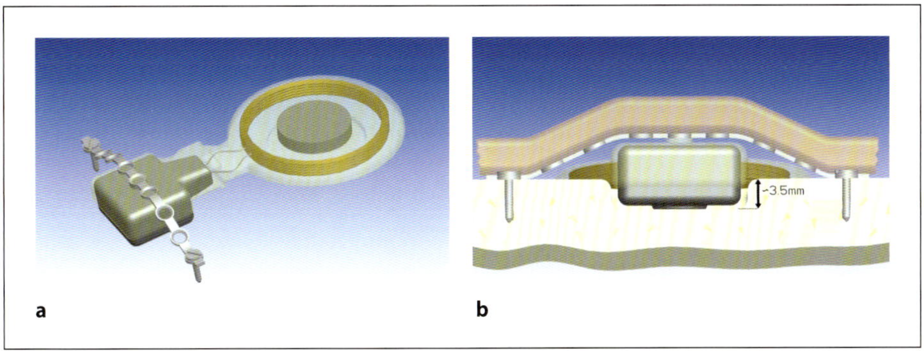

Fig. 5. The implanted part of the BCI consisting of a receiving coil, a retention magnet and the transducer (**a**) and the titanium transducer casing placed in a 3–4 mm deep recess of the skull bone, held in place and pressed against the skull bone by means of a titanium bar construction (**b**). The size of the transducer casing is approximately 11.5 × 13.5 × 6.5 mm.

attachment is used like in the Baha system. Also, using a screw attachment there must be a coupling arrangement between the bone-anchored fixture and the transducer casing to facilitate replacement of the transducer if needed for repair or an MRI investigation. Such coupling will also increase the depth of engagement in the temporal bone, maybe by a factor of two. To make the surgical procedure safe and simple, the depth of engagement in the temporal should be kept to a minimum. Instead, it is suggested for the BCI system that the casing should be pressed against the temporal bone and held in place with a standard craniofacial bar construction, as illustrated in figure 5. Hence, if replacement of the transducer is needed, the bar is released and the transducer can be easily removed. Thus, the engagement in the temporal bone can then be reduced to some 3–4 mm and the risk to damage deeper delicate structures will be very low.

If an MRI investigation has to be performed and the transducer is still in place, there is, according to preliminary tests, most likely no risk for the patient (forces were less than 2 N and the temperature increase was assumed negligible for a 1.5-tesla MRI procedure), but the transducer might be broken due to demagnetizations of biasing magnets. Images in the vicinity of the transducer (within 5–10 cm) will also be distorted. Further investigations are needed to more precisely determine adverse effects when an implanted transducer is in place during an MRI investigation. However, the standard procedure will probably be that the BCI system is temporarily removed if a patient requires an MRI investigation, and its attachment to the temporal bone is designed for such a procedure.

Design of the Implanted Transducer

A transducer for implantation in the skull bone must be hermetically capsulated in a titanium casing, which naturally means that this casing will be bigger than the transducer itself. Looking into the transducer used in Baha devices, and the normal anatomy of the temporal bone, one can easily conclude that they are too big. Therefore, a new transducer principle was developed called the Balanced Electromagnetic Separation Transducer (BEST). This new principle offers some advantages regarding size, output power and linearity that have been described by Håkansson [8].

Obviously, this transducer should be attached to the internal side of the casing which can be

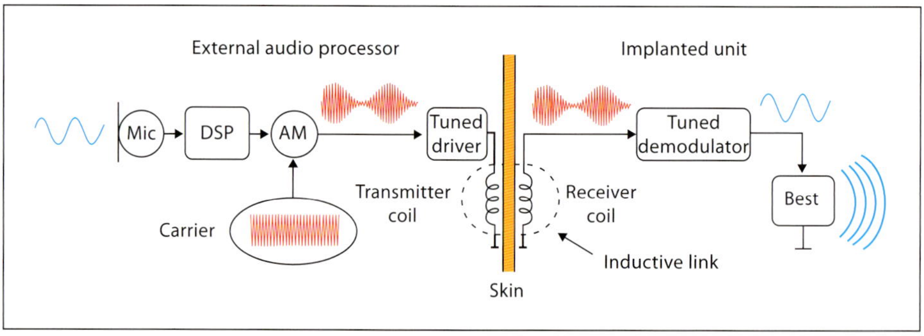

Fig. 6. Principle design of a full-scale BCI system. The skin-penetrating implant of the percutaneous Baha is here replaced by an amplitude modulation induction link including a carrier signal generator, a driver unit connected to a transmitting coil, an implanted receiving coil and a demodulator unit connected to the implanted transducer. Permanent magnets integrated in the coils for retention of the external unit are not shown.

done in different ways. In conventional Baha transducers, it is considered to be of utmost importance that the direct coupling to the skull bone should be done in a way that the transmission will not suffer from any sensitivity loss or cause distortion. This means that there will be one main resonance in Baha transducers, boosting the low frequency sensitivity (LF), see figure 2. Because of the inductive characteristic of the electrical input impedance, the HF range will have a roll-off by almost 20 dB per decade. However, it has also been pointed out that, from a clinical point of view, all present Baha should benefit from higher sensitivity and maximum power output (MPO) at higher frequencies [12, 13]. Therefore, the attachment of the BEST transducer to the casing in the BCI has been designed to improve the sensitivity and the MPO at higher frequencies. This is done by creating a second resonance in the HF range [18] (see figure 2). By adding a compliance when attaching the transducer to the casing, this HF resonance can be created without taking any extra space. The resonance is at present placed around 3 kHz, giving an HF sensitivity boost in the region of 2–5 kHz range. Above this resonance region, the roll-off will be increased as compared with the conventional Baha. If the resonance frequency is chosen to be 3 kHz, the crossing point where attenuation occurs is around 5 kHz, and hence this increased roll-off will have less consequence as it gives attenuation in a frequency region beyond where most speech information exists.

Design of the Sound Processor and the Induction Link

In order to keep the skin and subcutaneous tissues intact, the signal is transmitted through an inductive link to the implanted BEST transducer. The link consists of one external transmitting coil and one implanted receiving coil that are attached and aligned to each other with a permanent magnet retention system. As illustrated in figure 6, an amplitude modulation of the signal to a carrier frequency is needed to achieve an efficient transmission. Furthermore, both the driver and the receiver coils must be tuned to optimize the transmission through nominally 4–6 mm of soft tissues.

A BCI audio processor has been developed and is illustrated in figure 7. The BCI audio processor (left) looks very much like the Classic Baha as they have many common components, but here the transducer is replaced by a circular

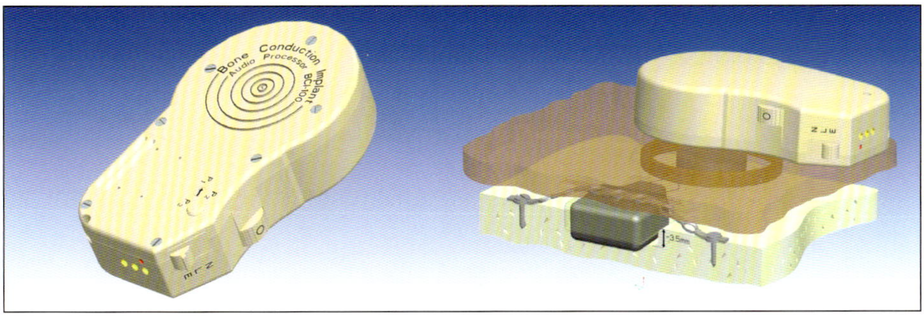

Fig. 7. The audio processor BCI-100 is based on a Baha casing where the transducer is replaced by a transmitting coil, a retention magnet and an induction link modulation and power electronics. The whole BCI system in situ is shown on the right.

transmitting coil and a magnet for retention. The power stage is driving the amplitude-modulated input signal according to the scheme illustrated in figure 6. This audio processor, called BCI-100, is regarded as an investigational device and it has all functionality but will be miniaturized in a later stage of the project. The whole BCI system in situ is shown in figure 7.

Preclinical Results

The whole BCI system has been tested under various conditions such as using a skull simulator [14], a dry skull, and in cadaver heads. Here a summary will be given of the results from a study on three embalmed cadavers by Håkansson et al. [18]. All cadavers had normal skull anatomy and were lying horizontally on a stainless steel table. One first fixture was placed in the standard Baha position in the parietal bone 55 mm behind the ear canal opening. A recess was then formed in the temporal bone just behind the ear canal for the attachment of the BCI transducer. In this chapter, these two positions are named 'Baha position' and 'BCI position'. These positions correspond to 'Pos A' and 'Pos B' respectively, in the paper by Håkansson et al. [18]. The casing of the BCI transducer was attached by using a clamping bar that was fixed by miniature orthopedic bone screws.

The sound processors used in this study comprised: (a) BCI, (b) Baha® Classic, (c) Baha Intenso. The BCI included a VSB® (Vibrant Med-El, Innsbruck, Austria) with factory preset gain and volume control (the VSB has no external controls). A laser doppler vibrometer (LDV) from Polytec (HLV-1000) was used to measure the vibration velocity of the cochlear promontory. The sound source was a stepped sine that was swept from 100 to 10,000 Hz. The sound field pressure levels presented to the microphone of the devices were kept constant at the following levels: 60, 70, and 90 dB SPL. The LDV output (velocity) was subsequently transferred to MatLab® where the promontory acceleration level was calculated.

The most important result in this study was the ipsilateral promontory acceleration responses (calculated from the measured velocity responses) at 90 dB SPL, also known to give the MPO of the devices. In figure 8, the difference in MPO obtained at the BCI position versus the typical Baha position are shown. It can be seen that the BCI position offers 0–10 dB improvement, varying over the frequency range from 700 to 7,000 Hz. In a similar way, the contralateral promontory responses were measured, but for these measurements it was found that the Baha position

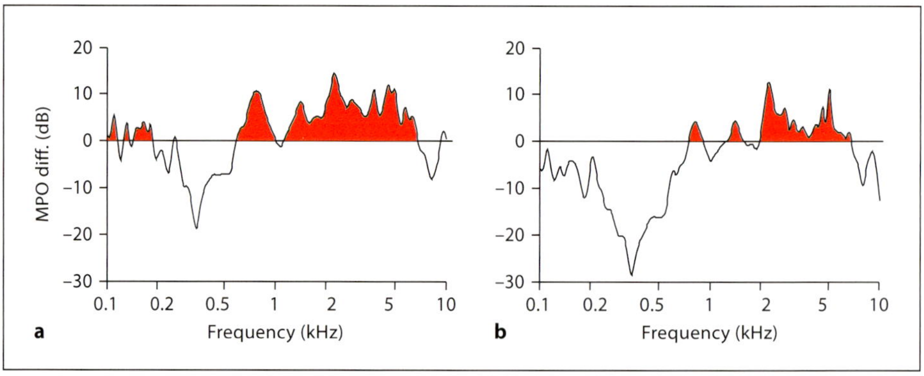

Fig. 8. Difference in ipsilateral MPO between the BCI system, and two well-known Baha sound processors: BCI vs. Baha Classic (**a**). BCI vs. Baha Intenso (**b**). The red area means that the BCI has a higher MPO than the Baha.

performed considerably better than in the BCI position.

Discussion

When comparing the 'acoustically' generated frequency responses between the different devices, only the MPO gives an adequate comparison of the potential capacity of the systems. At levels below the MPO, the response curves in each device can be changed by amplifier settings in a multitude of ways.

Considering all measurements, it seems that an implantable transducer can give an increased vibration level at the ipsilateral cochlear promontory compared with existing ear level Baha. One remaining uncertainty is whether this improvement in vibration level also implies an improvement in hearing. Psychoacoustic investigations are ongoing to address this question regarding interpretation of in vitro LDV responses at the promontory versus hearing perception. In one such investigation, subjects who have a Baha implant and also additional implants in the mastoid region for retaining an artificial outer ear were used. Preliminary results [Eeg-Olofsson, pers. commun.] indicate that a mastoid-positioned transducer (BCI position) gives a significantly better speech recognition as measured by the signal-to-noise ratio, than a parietal-positioned transducer (Baha position).

The potential hearing improvement with a BCI over a Baha should be balanced by the potential risk differences in the surgical procedures, as well as long-term effects. How this balance will turn out may differ between patients, and future in vivo studies are planned to clinically evaluate the whole BCI system in this respect.

It is also clear from these investigations that an SSD patient may not benefit from a BCI system since the present Baha system shows a significantly better transcranial transmission to the contralateral cochlea. On the other hand, this means that the sound transmission will be more directed to the ipsilateral cochlea when using the BCI system, and this finding can be beneficial for patients with bilateral implantation due to an improved possibility to extract binaural cues. It may also be beneficial to implant the BCI system on the hearing side of an SSD patient, and have a microphone on the deaf side, from which the signal is wirelessly transferred to the BCI. The improved HF response of the BCI transducer with the HF resonance may then be very useful for compensating the head shadow effect.

One other important question to address is: Why do we see this huge improvement in promontory response from 700 to 7,000 Hz when the excitation position moves from the Baha position to the BCI position? This is discussed in a little more detail by Håkansson et al. [18] and can be summarized as follows. The Baha is attached to a shell-like part of the parietal bone, whereas the BCI is attached to the mastoid and 'solid' portion of the temporal bone where the cochlea is situated. By increasing the frequency, the Baha position area of the skull bone is most likely elastically decoupled from the mastoid portion of the temporal bone, and hence there will be an increased attenuation by increasing frequency.

Finally, it was also found that the devices in the Baha position (especially the Intenso) were more prone to fall into oscillation at high gain settings as compared to the device in the BCI position. This is also probably due to the higher impedance of the bone in the BCI position compared to the bone in the Baha position.

Conclusions

There are many possibilities for improving BC devices in the future. Conventional BC devices can be improved by a better housing design and improved transducer technology, having the major advantage of being noninvasive and being a low-cost alternative. They are also an alternative for children below a certain age where Baha/BCI surgery is not appropriate.

Baha systems will most likely be improved by better fitting procedures of sound processors, and by developing more patient-optimized transducers, especially for single-sided deaf patients.

Alternative systems, like the Otomag system and the SoundBite system, may find a market position for certain patient groups with the major advantage of being less invasive than the Baha and BCI systems.

Implanted transducer systems, like the BCI system, have in preclinical studies shown to be a realistic alternative to a percutaneous Baha. These systems have the potential to meet the desires to achieve DBC stimulation and do not require permanent skin penetration. However, robust and long-term clinical human tests are needed before indications can be supported for these more invasive hearing systems.

Acknowledgement

The BCI project was supported by the Swedish agency for Innovation systems VINNOVA.

References

1 Håkansson B, Tjellström A, Rosenhall U, Carlsson P: The bone-anchored hearing aid: principle design and a psychoacoustical evaluation. Acta Otolaryngol 1985; 100:229–239.
2 Håkansson B, Lidén G, Tjellström A, Ringdahl A, Jacobsson M, Carlsson P, Erlandson BE: Ten years of experience with the Swedish bone-anchored hearing system. Ann Otol Rhinol Laryngol Suppl 1990;151:1–16.
3 Tjellström A, Håkansson B, Granström G: The bone-anchored hearing aids – current status in adults and children. Otolaryngol Clin North Am 2001;34:337–364.
4 Håkansson B: Technical development of the BAHA – a historical review covering the first twenty years. Firmly Anchored, Baha Users Support (Kent) 2006;17. http://www.baha-users-support.com/birth_of_baha.php.
5 Hodgetts WE: Other implantable devices: bone-anchored hearing aids; in Seewald R, Tharpe AM: Comprehensive Handbook of Pediatric Audiology. San Diego, Plural Publishing, 2010, chapter 28.
6 Snik AF, Mylanus EA, Proops DW, Wolfaardt JF, Hodgetts WE, Somers T, Niparko JK, Wazen JJ, Sterkers O, Cremers CW, Tjellström A: Consensus statements on the BAHA system: where do we stand at present? Ann Otol Rhinol Laryngol Suppl 2005;195:2–12.
7 Raicevich G, Burwood E, Dillon H: Taking the pressure off bone conduction hearing aid users. Aust N Z J Audiol 2008;30:113–118.
8 Håkansson B: The balanced electromagnetic separation transducer – a new bone conduction transducer. J Acoust Soc Am 2003;113:818–825.

9 Hough J, Vernon J, Dormer K, et al: Experiences with implantable hearing devices and a presentation of a new device. Ann Otol Rhinol Laryngol 1986; 95:60–65.
10 Håkansson B, Tjellström A, Carlsson P: Percutaneous vs transcutaneous transducers for hearing by direct bone conduction. Otolaryngol Head Neck Surg 1990;102:339–344.
11 Siegert R: Die magnetische Ankopplung von Knochenleitungshörgeräten ohne offene Implantate – Prinzip und erste Ergebnisse einer neuen Knochenleitungsversorgung. Laryngo-Rhino-Otol 2010;89:346–351.
12 Hodgetts WE, Hagler P, Hakansson B, Soli S: Technology-limited and patient-derived versus audibility-derived fittings in Baha users: a validation study. Ear Hear 2010;31:1-x.
13 Hodgetts WE, Håkansson BE, Hagler Pl, Soli S: A comparison of three approaches to verifying aided Baha output. Int J Audiol 2010;49:286–295.
14 Håkansson B, Carlsson P: Skull simulator for direct bone conduction hearing devices. Scand Audiol 1989;18:91–98.
15 Håkansson B, Carlsson P: Arrangement in a hearing aid device. US patent 4,904, 233, 1990.
16 Håkansson B: Percutaneous bone anchored transferring device. US patent 6,840,919, 2005.
17 Håkansson B, Eeg-Olofsson M, Reinfeldt S, Stenfelt S, Granström G: Percutaneous versus transcutaneous bone conduction implant system: a feasibility study on a cadaver head. Otol Neurotol 2008;29: 1132–1139.
18 Håkansson B, Reinfeldt S, Eeg-Olofsson M, Östli P, Taghavi H, Adler J, Gabrielsson J, Stenfelt S, Granström G: A novel bone conduction implant (BCI) – engineering aspects and preclinical studies. Int J Audiology 2010;49:203–215.
19 Eeg-Olofsson M, Granström G, Stenfelt S, Tjellström A: Transmission of bone-conducted sound in the human skull measured by cochlear vibrations. Int J Audiol 2008;47:1–9.
20 Reinfeldt S, Östli P, Håkansson B, Stenfelt S: Hearing one's own voice during phoneme vocalization – transmission by air and bone conduction. J Acoust Soc Am 2010;128:751–762.
21 Stenfelt S, Håkansson B: Sensitivity to bone-conducted sound: excitation of the mastoid vs the teeth. Scand Audiol 1999; 28:190–198.
22 Popelka GR, Derebery J, Blevins NH, Murray M, Moore BCJ, Sweetow RW, Wu B, Katsis M: Preliminary evaluation of a novel bone-conduction device for single-sided deafness. Otol Neurotol 2010;31: 492–497.

Bo Håkansson
Chalmers University of Technology, Department of Signals and Systems
SE–412 96 Göteborg (Sweden)
Tel. +46 31 772 18, Fax +46 31 772 1782, E-Mail boh@chalmers.se

Author Index

Subject Index